Revolutionary
Spiritual Healing

Revolutionary Spiritual Healing

Sondra Ray

with
Markus Ray

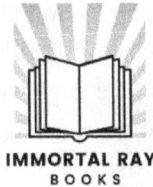

IMMORTAL RAY
BOOKS

Other Books by Sondra Ray

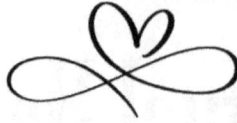

- The Only Diet There Is
- Rebirthing in the New Age
- I Deserve Love
- Loving Relationships I
- Celebration of Breath
- Ideal Birth
- Drinking the Divine
- Pure Joy
- Inner Communion
- How to Be Chic, Fabulous, and Live Forever
- Interlude with the Gods
- Loving Relationships II
- Essays on Creating Sacred Relationships
- Healing and Holiness
- Pele's Wish
- Relationships Treasury
- Rock Your World with the Divine Mother
- Liberation Breathing: The Divine Mother's Gift
- Spiritual intimacy: What You Really Want with a Mate
- Babaji: My Miraculous Meetings with a Maha Avatar
- Liberation: Freedom from Your Biggest Block to Pure Joy
- The New Loving Relationships Book
- I Deserve Love (2nd Edition)
- Physical Immortality: How to Overcome Death
- The Perfection of Babaji
- Lately I've Been Thinking I
- Lately I've Been Thinking II
- The Supermarket for a Meaningful Life
- Outside the Box with Babaji

IMMORTAL RAY PRODUCTIONS
301 TINGEY STREET SE, #302
WASHINGTON DC, 20003

immortalrayproductions@gmail.com

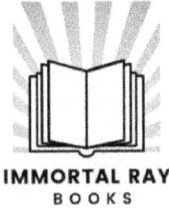

IMMORTAL RAY
B O O K S

Library of Congress Cataloging in Publication Data

Ray, Sondra; Revolutionary Spiritual Healing

1. Self-Help 2. Spiritual Healing 3. Life-Wisdom

Cover Design: Immortal Ray Productions
Front Cover Painting: Kriss Guenzati Dubini

ISBN 13: Paperback | 978-1-950684-20-5

ISBN 13: Hardback | 978-1-950684-21-2

ISBN 13: E-Book | 978-1-950684-22-9

Dedication

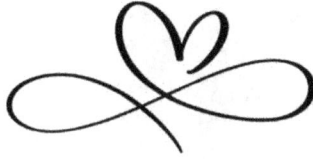

To my masters Babaji, Ammachi, and Jesus. This is our "Dream Team" and they have released me from every condition I have had. THANK YOU FOREVER!

To Markus, my husband, best friend, and spiritual partner who has expanded my creativity, supported my projects, helped me perfect and heal myself, advanced my enlightenment, encouraged me in every crisis, and enabled me to express my divinity with him as we serve together in bliss and peace.

And to Ethel, my mother, who allowed me to be different, taught me very high thoughts, and grounded me in strength and who even now assists Markus and me from the other side in our current work.

This book is titled *Revolutionary Spiritual Healing* because of its alignment with A Course in Miracles which itself is a totally revolutionary approach to life, living, and spiritual transformation. Revolutionary, too, because it brings to light the fact that the personal lies and unconscious death urge we carry create illness and death. I know of no other books on this subject.

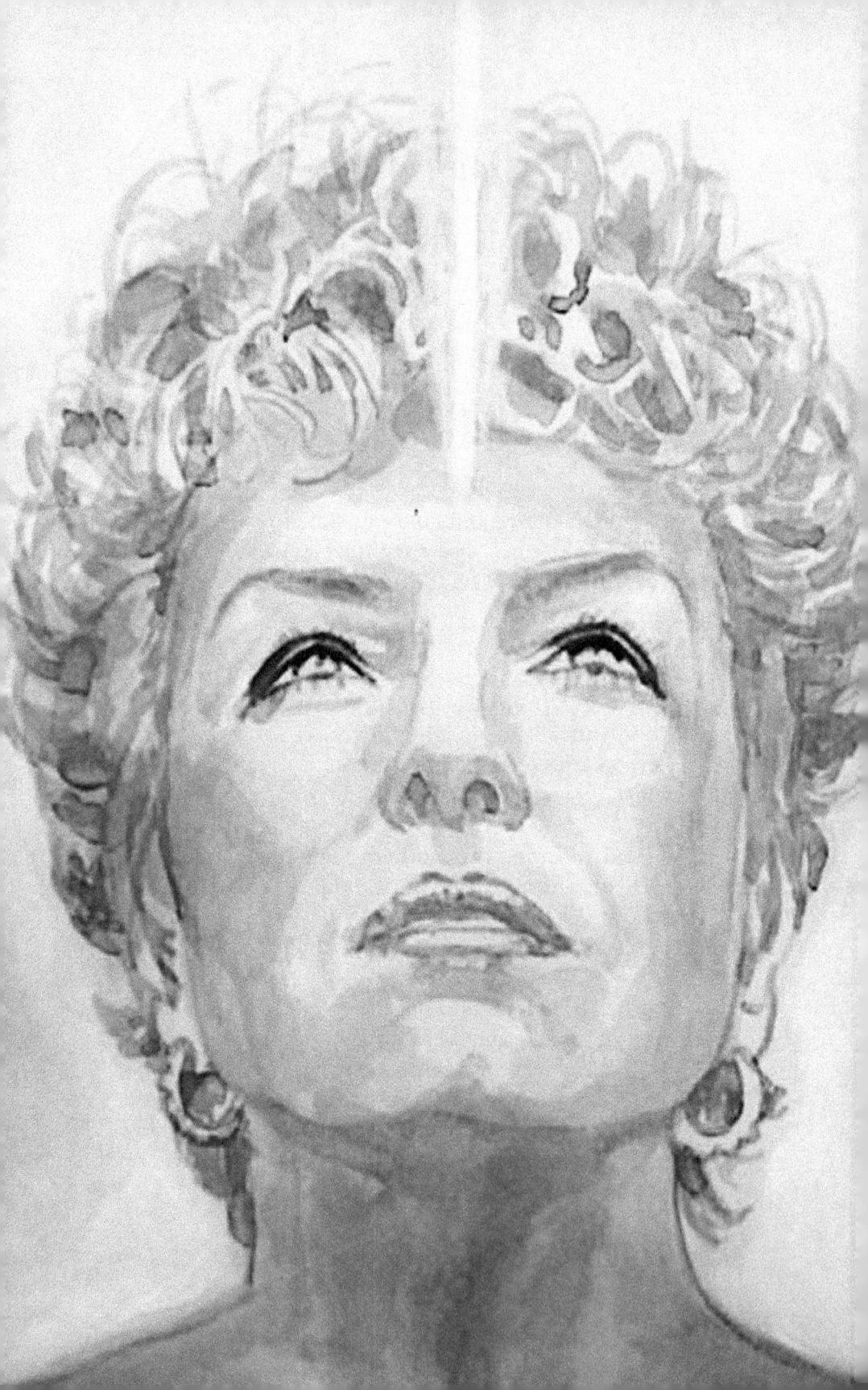

Sickness is a defense against the truth.

When I am healed, I am not healed alone.

Lessons #136 & #137 in A Course in Miracles

Contents

Foreword

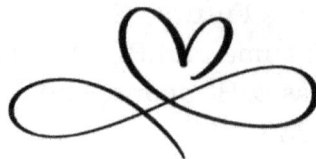

Are you willing to do whatever it takes to be completely healed of any negative condition in your life? This book is about taking complete responsibility for our health—of body, mind and spirit. We rule our mind, which in turn rules our body. What Sondra Ray shows us over and over again is that we are ultimately responsible for our illnesses and all the things in our life that need healing. It is revolutionary in this sense: within us in the "cause" for all disease, and with the right perspective, within us is also the cure for all disease. We are the ones who made up our diseases, and we are the ones who can unmake them. This level of responsibility and healing, extending all the way into the spiritual realms of our being, can truly be called "revolutionary."

I met Sondra Ray in 1985. Two things that she said back then stirred me up to take more responsibility for the content of my mind. One was, "Your thought is creative." Nothing happens to me, including all disease, that is not a result of some thought I have, either subconscious or conscious. That statement began my long process of taking true responsibility for everything that happens in my life. After that I was not able to pretend to be a "victim" of anything. The other thing she said was, "A Course in Miracles is the most important book written in 2000 years." That statement prompted me to begin a serious study of that work for the next 35 plus years, which I continue to this day—and for the rest of my life. Those two statements were revolutionary for me. They have continued to unfold in my life to this day, which have brought incredible gratitude to my soul.

Sondra has written 30 books on the subjects of Healing, Relationships, Ideal Birth, Spirituality, and Rebirthing / Breathwork which she helped pioneer since 1974 all over the world. She has also written about Spiritual Connection and Communion, The Divine Mother, A Course in Miracles, Babaji, the "Yogi Christ" of India in the spiritual genre. Some of her most important work in the psychological genre concerns how our birth trauma and "personal lies" replay and affect our relationships. How do these early birth traumas cause sabotaging experiences in our life? She was a Nurse Practitioner for 14 years prior to her metaphysical directions. She used her medical knowledge as a springboard to discover the more subtle causes and sub-consciousness factors contributing to our "dis-eases."

This book is about all of what she discovered. It is an extension and rewrite of her former book, *Healing and Holiness,* that she published twenty years ago with Celestial Arts. Some parts of this book are reiterations of the most important points she wrote about when she crossed her 61st year back then. Other parts are new altogether. This book is conceived and written in a new vibration. Now Sondra Ray has celebrated her 81st birthday, and the vitality of her philosophy and practice of Physical Immortality is more tempered and tested. With age comes wisdom, but also with age comes the challenge more poignantly of overcoming our *unconscious death urge.*

The collective *planned obsolescence* of the body/mind is a force to be reckoned with. The "mental gravity" of negative thinking more urgently needs our attention to reverse the march of "old age." Undoing our conditioning around death is more crucial the older we get. If we truly want to live a vital and productive life after sixty-five, this book offers that to a mature audience. If we want to start a longevity path in our thirties it gives millennials that too. What we learn in this book is a *love of correction* starting right now, whatever our age, so consequences of modern stresses do not accumulate and eventually get the better of us through disease and ultimate death.

Sondra Ray gives us a solution to aging, sickness and death in *Revolutionary Spiritual Healing*. Reading her stories about her own health challenges and how she overcame them with spiritual practices inspires us to do the same. A spiritual solution to our problems is what is needed in this highly "scientific" age. Getting our "heads straight" that we are the rulers of our life in all aspects of body, mind and spirit puts us in the driver's seat of our own healing process. The "healer" is the mind of the patient himself.

Taking this journey of healing with Sondra Ray will shed light on your own. You will think of "disease" differently—not as some unfortunate force of nature that got the better of you, but a result of thought patterns and behaviors you can change. *Revolutionary Spiritual Healing* is nothing short of the miracle of taking responsibility 100% for your whole Life. What is fully alive and connected to its Divine Source cannot see death. Life is inevitable, not death. God in this book will make that truth apparent.

—Markus Ray

Preface

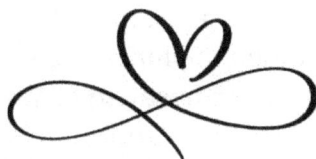

My master Babaji told those of us who had come to India, "I could heal you all instantly, but what would you learn?"

We had to learn to work out our problems by ourselves. Of course, we learned more quickly with Babaji's support, and He often took pity on us and took on some of our karma to lighten our loads. With and without Babaji's guidance, I have had my share of "learning experiences," most of which I do not care to repeat. And while I have been good at helping others heal themselves, I have not always been good at healing myself. It is because of this that I believe I have learned so much!

I have been a healer since day one, but I was hesitant to write a book on this subject until I felt myself reasonably well healed. In truth, until we are all like Jesus and Babaji, we have something to clear. So, the process goes on.

A real miracle occurred at my birth—my grandfather was instantly healed of a depression at the sight of me—but I always felt I had failed because of my father's death. He was sick and in and out of hospitals my entire childhood. Watching him slowly die, day-by-day, was devastating. Why couldn't I save him? My preoccupation with healing had begun. I often helped care for him, starting at three years old, and when I was six, I told him exactly how to heal himself! That was too much of a shock for my family, and they reprimanded me for being so presumptuous. I held myself back a lot because of that.

I became a nurse to understand why people get sick and die, but I did not find the answers in Western medicine that I intuitively sought. I wanted to see permanent healing, not the same symptoms recurring in patients who returned to hospitals again and again. I desperately wanted to know how to prevent disease and death.

I was taught that the Bible says ". . . with God all things are possible." I took this promise literally and believed that as a child of God I deserved to know how to be permanently healed and how to live forever!

What disturbed me most about my father's chronic illness and death was that modern medicine and religion failed him. He died and I did not understand why. Later, modern medicine and religion failed my sister, who died of melanoma. And they failed me as well. I endured continuous physical pain for twelve to fourteen years after my father died. Modern Western medicine could not help me, so I began searching for other answers.

Finally, I was able to begin a real journey of self-healing while experiencing everything possible using alternative methods. My life became a great transition away from the addiction to Western medicine. I have studied with many healers whose various techniques taught me something new about healing. Healers are my dearest colleagues; I have a special affinity for them and their quiet, hard work in all parts of the world. Many of them are unacknowledged for their important spiritual service to humanity, and I want to acknowledge all of them now.

I have basically reconditioned myself about what *healing* really means. A Course in Miracles states that "truth cannot deal with errors that we want to keep." Why we want to keep our errors rather than to be healed is a deep subject. We may think we want to be healed, but our unconscious sabotage patterns are stronger than we realize. Our challenge is to understand how the unconscious mind works and learn how to change it.

Revolutionary Spiritual Healing is for those who truly want to be permanently healed and for those who want to help others discover how to do the same. It is an attempt to share with others what I have learned thus far in my healing journey, but it is not my last word on this subject. I am still improving. A great teacher is there to save you time. It took me over fifty years to learn all that is in this book. I am certain that it will save you lots of time.

This book is slanted to healing physical conditions. However, a great deal of the information and prayers will also apply to healing emotional and other conditions in your life.

Sometimes you will notice that things are repeated. This is deliberate. It means the point is super important!

—Sondra Ray

Introduction

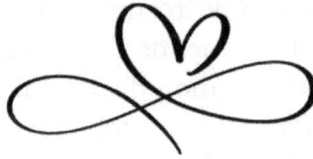

Revolutionary Spiritual Healing takes us beyond the known channels of treating our "ailments" with physical or even mental substances, into different realms of power and potential for correcting our errors. We need a different way of looking at "sickness" and the "healing of sickness." Sickness is an error, in the view that perfect health and happiness are our natural states of being. Anything but supreme joy is a deviation from the essence of our being. Perfect health is our natural state of being.

You can defend the duality of an apparent *human condition,* but we will have to face, sooner or later, that we are responsible for those conditions, and we "make them up" as we go along in the creation of our "life." The mind rules us in the end. And what is "in our mind" is at the root of these conditions. And we cannot heal without taking 100% responsibility for all thoughts, words, deeds and actions we have projected upon ourselves from the beginning of time immemorial. There is a "cause and effect" of thought, call it "karma" if you will, but we cannot escape this law of manifestation: what one thinks about expands and attracts a result. Thought is never "idle," and negative thoughts will inevitably produce painful and negative results. Ill health is a result of ill thinking. All true healing must correct the disease at the level where it was made, and that involves a rebooting of the mind to a more-healthy state of original perfection.

Sondra Ray is my consort. I have been with her 24/7/365 for 15 years now. I have learned some things about her that I would like to share here. She is all about her Mission. She is all about *Revolutionary Spiritual Healing.* She is all about the New Paradigm of Joy in Relationships. She is all about the Divine Mother's Power to heal us of everything "off" in our physical & mental dimension, and the Divine Father's Power to heal us of everything "off" in our spiritual dimension. She represents a complete package. She is even dedicated to seeing that "death itself" is a function of consciousness. When we think a certain way, we get old, sick, wither away, and die. When we think a different way, and truly connect with the Divine Forces within us, we heal and live indefinitely, even rejuvenating our "physical body" to a state of being that is unaffected by time, and the entropic forces of physical decay. This is what she would call *Revolutionary Spiritual Healing.*

It has some prerequisites. Without them, one can miss the point altogether, and reading this book will not enact the inner transformation of healing in you that it has the potential to enact. You will block it, in other words. First, we all have to start with the fact that all pain and sickness we experience in life is "self-inflicted." Be it consciously inflicted, or unconsciously inflicted, it is still a result of our minds and what is in our minds.

Some cutting-edge scientists realize what is subconsciously held in our mind is proportionally massive, when set against our conscious awareness. And this huge subconscious mass of memory is producing results in our life that may seem to "come out of nowhere." This includes all of the self-sabotaging thoughts we call "personal lies," such as "I am not good enough," "I am wrong," "I am unlovable," "I am not wanted," and simply, "I don't want to be here" in this life of mine I have made up for myself. The nature of thought itself seems to have this built-in "worst critic" of negativity. We have become a culture of narcissists and bi-polar self-promoters— isolated, as it seems, in an ocean of social media. Going on with survival as we know it is not bringing peace of mind, or a sense of well-being, or ultimately supreme happiness. Why not? We are as equipped as ever to be the masters of our own destiny.

Supreme happiness, as anything "supreme," is an absolute, not a "relative" state. Certain laws are immutable. When it comes to those states deemed ultimately desirable, such as Love, Gratitude, Equanimity, Joy, Satisfaction, Happiness, Honesty, Truth, etc. we find they ascend above the duality of thought. They are states of being without opposites when fully realized. And I could say my life together with Sondra Ray has the sole responsibility to forgive all our lower states of relative being, in order to embrace and apply our Higher States of Absolute Being. "Love is not love, which alters, when alteration finds," said Shakespeare. True Love has no opposite, in other words. It is not "counterbalanced" by "hate." At the level of the Absolute, there is no "hate." At the level of the Absolute, there is no "sickness." And this is where *Revolutionary Spiritual Healing* wants to take us. But we must forgive ourselves completely of indulging in lower states of consciousness, or I should say "unconsciousness," that produced our problems and illnesses in the first place.

The Power of Love can heal absolutely, but we have to make contact with its absolute version that has no "opposite." Rising above the duality of thought as we know it will take a lot of attention. But manifesting pain and suffering takes a lot of attention as well. So, which would we rather have—our version of a polite "hell" we made up, or a God-Given Heaven that is our original State of Being in which we were created? This "return to the Absolute" is *Revolutionary Spiritual Healing.*

Without the boon of the Divine Mother, transformation into our absolute Immortal Being is not possible. Sondra was told this by her Master Teachers. What does it really mean? How do we receive that boon? What is the Divine Mother exactly, and how do we make contact with Her and maintain this contact? Most Western models of religious belief seem to be heavily biased toward a Masculine God who metes out a final judgment in the end of whether our life here on earth was meritorious for receiving a Heaven in our "afterlife." The Divine Mother, the Life Force that makes the planets, stars, and cosmos itself out of endless elements, seems to have no say in our Destiny of Being. Our Ideal Being is separated, it seems, from an incarnate existence.

This book, *Revolutionary Spiritual Healing,* questions that separation. If you are reading this, you have a body. You have a mind full of thoughts. You have a language, English, that you know and we can therefore communicate. You have a yearning to heal, or you would not have picked up this book in the first place. We do not want to waste your time, nor ours. So here is the crux of it. The Divine Mother is a Life Force pulsing in you. You are never separated from Her, just as you are never separated from the Spirit of the Father. Your Spirit-Mind-and Body are ONE BEING all working in perfect harmony. And this harmony is Health and Immortality. You are that in truth. This book is to restore your awareness of that Truth. It is Simple. It is Loving. It is the greatest Service you can render to yourself and others. To rise to the height of your True Self is the action of *Revolutionary Spiritual Healing.* You can do this by reading this book. May it start you on a journey that is already completed. May it awaken you to Greater Happiness. May it heal you of all that ails you now, or will ever cause you discomfort in the future. May it be your ultimate release from all suffering, in all time and space, forever.

I *re-present* to you Sondra Ray. I present to you her latest book in her Divine Mission of traveling the High Road. I present to you *Revolutionary Spiritual Healing.*

LOVE,

MARKUS RAY
Washington DC
August 4, 2023

Revolutionary Spiritual Healing

1.

Healing Myself

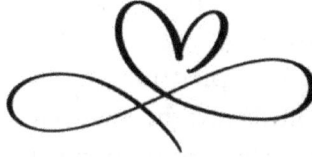

I could have healed myself more quickly had I known at the time of my "illnesses" all the information that is in this book, especially what I have recently discovered about prayer techniques. You could say that I traveled the "low road" of trial, error, and struggle. This chapter is about that low road when I was addicted to the Western medical models. And yet, I learned so much. Remember, I became a nurse and was conditioned by the conventional system. I was afraid to let go of that system. I thought I needed doctors to survive, and it was that dependence that kept me in weakness and helplessness. As you will see, even after I began to give up those Western methods of healing and to explore alternative methods, I was still addicted to struggle. I made my healing process more difficult than necessary, and I wasted a lot of time worrying I would never get over some of those symptoms. My constant worry considerably slowed down the healing process.

When I finally became disenchanted with my own medical profession, I left it to study spiritual healing. However, even after I left, I was not free; I was just rebelling. I became arrogant and canceled my medical insurance. I went without insurance for ten full years to prove that I would never need a doctor again. But my attitude was not right, and eventually my arrogance caught up with me. I had a very humbling experience that forced me to go back and forgive "modern" western medicine for not healing my father. It took me over a decade to wean myself from the system. I practiced spiritual self-healing as much as possible, but I still sought medical doctors on a couple of occasions. Realizing that totally mastering self-healing would be a long process, I tried to be patient with myself.

Although this book is about how to heal spiritually without the addiction to modern medicine, there may be times when your fear of giving up traditional methods is too great to overcome. In those cases, you need to go to a doctor. A few years ago, I fell in the middle of the night and broke a bone in my shoulder, and needed an MD surgeon to fix it. I am not at the point I can instantly heal a broken bone, although there are some Kahuna healers who have mastered this. I still had to process myself on why I attracted this "incident." But, in the long run, do not limit yourself to traditional methods alone. Try other techniques of healing. Before running to a doctor, you may want to try some of the techniques discussed in this book. The goal is self-healing, and PREVENTION of disease is the ultimate goal.

I am not proud of all the illnesses and negative physical conditions I have manifested over the years, and I wish that learning had been easier. Perhaps the sharing of my healing journey will help others come through their own physical and spiritual healing much faster.

The temptation to get sick was always very strong in our house, as well as in our small Iowa town of three hundred. It seemed that people were dying right and left. The worst part of it was that we children were required to march to the cemetery every time someone died. I took those deaths seriously because everyone in my town was my "family" in one sense or another.

When I was five, I asked my Sunday School teacher why they died. She said, "The Lord took them away." I questioned further, "Does that mean God kills people?" She did not answer me. She remained silent. This haunted me for much of my life and as a result I rebelled. (If God killed my father, how can I be a Christian?) I ended up marrying an atheist the first time because of this.

My father was sick most of the time, in and out of hospitals. I loved my father and wanted to be like him, but I did not want to be sick. So, it was a tricky relationship for me. When he was twelve, my dad apparently had rheumatic fever. Later he died of rheumatic heart disease. When he was in the hospital in neighboring Mason City, Iowa, the nuns never let me in to see him because I was not "old enough." (Can you believe they would not let kids in to see their parents?) He was always there for a long time, so I used to sneak up the fire escape, crawl through the window, and sit with him on the hospital bed. He got better when he saw me. We usually had just a few minutes together before I was discovered. My dad used to say to the nuns, "You leave her alone." But they threw me out just the same. Why is it that the medical profession didn't realize that children can be healers for their parents?

When I was twelve, I developed the same symptoms of rheumatic fever as my father. I got very sick. The doctors could not find any spirochetes or anything else abnormal in my blood. They told my mother that I had a "pseudo" case—my illness wasn't real. Obviously, I was "empathizing" with my father.

My Cat Ashram

I used to have about 40 cats outside that I would relate to. They followed me everywhere except when I rode my bike to town. We had huge yards, many barns, and chicken houses. That was great for the cats and all their litters. Different mother cats had different litters here and there and somehow, I was in charge of them all (at least I thought so). My cats kept me going. If I felt bad, I could talk to my cats. They sat on the lawn and patiently listened to me while I gave them long lectures and shared my feelings. (It was perfect practice for being a public speaker later as they never interrupted me, walked out, or looked bored!) I always felt better after these sessions, and as a child, I was rarely sick except for that one false alarm. I simply did not have time to think about getting sick. I was busy with my cats!

At night, when my dad and grandpa walked out to the pasture to milk the cows, they deliberately clanged the milk pails together, and all the cats came running. It was like a big parade! My dad and grandpa played a game with my cats, aiming the cow's teat, full of milk, at a certain cat's mouth. The cats liked this game, and I learned to milk the cows the same way.

Every hay season, my grandpa came over to our house, opened the door, and yelled, "Sondie, there is a new litter of kittens in the hay barn." Then he shut the door and headed for the hayloft. I ran after him as fast as I could and climbed up the wooden slats to the loft. So many hay bales were always piled up in so many ways that it took me a long time to find the new litter. It was exciting beyond belief when I finally found them.

Sometimes I felt that certain cats were not very good mothers, and in such cases, when they ignored their young, I had wet nurses on the side. Blackie was the best surrogate mother, and she was always willing to nurse kittens that I felt were ignored by other mothers. When Blackie died, old and blind, I was devastated. I held a major funeral for her, and all the cats had to attend. After all, that was the way it was done in our town!

I remember a picture of myself taken on one of my birthdays. My mom had put my angel-food cake on the sidewalk, and the cats came and licked off the frosting. My hair was in long curls with green bows on the top, and the photo reminds me of how I shared everything with my cats.

One day my grandpa gave me a big tent and my dad built a wooden floor for it and put in electricity. I had a big bed in there, and I was in heaven because I could sleep with my cats! I was out there even during heavy rainstorms. Blackie always had top priority and got to sleep by my face. She was, after all, the best mother and "healer" of my cat family.

My cats were my gurus and my healers when I was young. They took care of me, and I took care of them. Even after I went off to college, my cats waited for me to come home.

The most amazing thing happened to me when I got older and became a successful writer. My publishers produced a book called *Why Cats Paint*. Phil, the owner of the publishing company, had so much fun doing that book—almost as much fun as I had as a kid with my cats. He even had a display in the gallery below the publishing house of live cats painting while people watched. Apparently, certain cats really do love to paint.

I was pretty happy as a kid (except for my dad's illness). I used to ride my bike around and visit the sick people in town and try to cheer them up.

Trouble Begins

When I went to college and left home and my cat ashram, trouble with my physical conditions began. My father had just died. He died the night before I was to graduate with honors from high school. I was salutatorian, having missed being valedictorian by one point. The salutatorian was required to give the traditional "Message to the Parents" lecture. Everyone in town was in the audience, all three hundred. They all knew my father had just died. I tried to give a tribute to my dad. I was devastated and frozen in grief. I have no idea what I said. Everyone in the audience was crying. My graduation turned into another funeral!

So began a long string of negative physical conditions, and I was forced to deal with issues of health and healing on a very dramatic level. I did not know why I created so many illnesses in my body during the following years. I thought maybe it was because I had always been around sick people as a child, and I had been unconsciously programmed to repeat the pattern. I thought maybe I had a lot of past-life karma or something. I thought maybe I was full of anger toward God about death and dying issues. I thought maybe my strong ego needed to be tamed. I thought maybe my mission in life was to become a healer and master the art of self-healing, so this was how I had to learn. Later I found out that my "unconscious death urge" was activated when my father died. Of course, I did not understand that at the time. That I will explain later.

In my adult life, I have created the following illnesses: insomnia, fourteen years of migrating pains, severe hair loss, severe food neurosis, acute arthritis, severe sinusitis, acute hypothermia, melanoma, severe gastritis, anorexia, rheumatism, paralysis over my heart chakra, a few near-death experiences, and a few other various and sundry ailments. I healed these conditions mostly with my mind and alternative methods, except on two occasions when I was so afraid that I lost my faith in spiritual healing. On those two occasions, I turned to modern medicine, but I eventually realized that my fear had great power over my physical health. My life has been one healing lesson after another, and I hope this book will be of value to others who are on the same journey of self-healing and physical immortality. I have learned, and I believe, that all illnesses—even death—are conditions that human beings have created for one reason or another. My healing journey has led me closer to understanding the source of these conditions.

Insomnia

After my father died, I left for my freshman year in college. I was determined to take pre-med and become a nurse, and I was determined to make straight A's. I had a scholarship to Augustana College, a Lutheran church college in Sioux Falls, South Dakota. At Augustana, the students were required to attend service at the chapel every day. All I could do was stand outside the chapel and cry. I never could go inside. And I could not sleep. I was afraid to shut my eyes; afraid I would wake up dead. (I know that sounds funny!) In other words, I really believed I would die in my sleep, so I simply did not sleep. I rarely told anyone about my condition. No one would have believed it anyway because I still managed to get straight A's. I was always trying to prove myself.

Finally, insomnia had taken its toll and I began to experience high fevers. I was put in a local hospital, and the college called my mother. The doctors told her they could not find anything wrong with me whatsoever. Once again, I seemed to be manifesting another psychosomatic illness. (Later I would learn that *all* illness is *mental* illness.) The doctors asked us both if we were willing for me to go into therapy. I had one therapy session with a psychiatrist who put me under hypnosis. After the session, he informed both my mother and me that I was not disturbed enough to warrant his high fees. (Bless his honest heart!) He suggested that I might need group therapy to share with other people my feelings about my father's death.

Off to group therapy I went. I did okay with it for a while until one of the men, a minister's son, asked me out for a date. He took me to see the movie *Suddenly Last Summer* starring Elizabeth Taylor.

Tennessee Williams is intense. During the movie my date was gripping the arms of the seat. When the movie ended, he informed me that he was going back in to see it again, leaving me standing there alone. So much for my first date in college. The next day he was admitted to a psychiatric ward! I went to visit him and his father, the minister, was there. *So much for religion* I thought. Religion had failed again, and I was really confused.

That summer I worked as a waitress at the Stanley Hotel in Estes Park, Colorado. Keeping busy and serving others healed me. Apparently, four thousand applications had been submitted by college students, and only thirty were hired by the hotel. I had not completed an application, but got the personnel staff's attention by sending a letter explaining why they should hire me. (Even though I was an emotional mess, my Higher Self was working. Who wants to sort through four thousand applications?) That letter worked and I got the job! Once I started to have fun and become more comfortable with sharing my feelings, I quickly got over insomnia.

Amoebic Dysentery and Cystitis

I finally rebelled, left the church school, and went off to the University of Florida College of Nursing. I went there for two reasons: First, I could get summers off, which allowed me to work to pay college expenses. Next, it was one of the biggest party schools in the nation (according to *Playboy* magazine). I was fed up with the religious and medical dogma of the Midwest. I needed to relax and have some fun! To be able to attend classes in Bermuda shorts was mind-blowing. I felt I had experienced a miracle.

In a short time, I met a young man who became my husband, a real genius and adventurer. He was an atheist—perfect for me at the time. I did not understand the dynamics of it all then, but I was angry with God about my father's long illness and death. I was in love, and we married right after my graduation. We were both inspired by President Kennedy to join the Peace Corps and were part of the first 10 groups that went abroad. You could say it was my boot camp training into world service. Our first assignment was Peru. I was very happy, and we both felt we were rebelling against the established norms and making a real difference in the world at the same time. To travel and serve others was a dream come true. We had a big shock as we landed in Peru. The pilot informed us that President Kennedy had just been shot and killed. We were devastated to say the least. We had no time to process this however. We were immediately assigned to give typhoid shots in a barrio.

Our assignment in Chimbote was tough and in an area that almost never saw rain. Squatter settlements were everywhere. Our hut had no roof per se, only a makeshift pole-and-straw cover. There was no electricity, no running water, and no indoor plumbing. People relieved themselves in the street in front of everyone. It did not bother me that much to see men peeing in the street in front of our hut, but to see them with their pants pulled down, squatting, was another thing. (At least the women were covered by their long skirts). Just to cook healthy meals was an ordeal. I had to pressure-cook everything on the primus stove. It was a real adventure, for sure, and I was determined to see it through.

Before long, we both developed amoebic dysentery despite our preventive efforts. We used to lay in bed and analyze which of us had the worst cramps and diarrhea. Even though we had been prepared for the possibility of this illness, blood in our stools was a scary thing, even for a nurse. Eventually, my husband lost his hair. He had developed a much rarer and stronger form of the amoeba.

I was not prepared for an attack of severe pain in my kidneys and blood in my urine. It was like urinating razor blades. I recognized the symptoms from my nursing books: honeymoon cystitis. It was excruciating. One did not dare consider going to a hospital in that town. The beds had no sheets and filth was everywhere. I had been taking care of babies in that hospital in the worst conditions and had seen many of them die of illness and starvation. Plague epidemics were on the rise. My husband wired Lima. A Peace Corps helicopter came to evacuate me.

Word got out that I was really sick. I did not think I was so sick at the time. I had IVs and thought I was going to be fine. Many of the Peace Corps volunteers heard I was dying and left their posts to visit me. I recovered, but the condition continued and became more chronic later. Often during my marriage, my condition was so bad that I ended up hospitalized, needing dilation and other treatments. Sometimes I had to stay on Macrodantin for a year at a time. I became afraid of sex. It ruined our sex life. The medical profession could not cure me of this condition. I was a nurse, but I had no idea of alternative healing methods.

My husband and I divorced partly over that. After my divorce, I began to have fewer problems with cystitis even with more sexual experiences. THAT was odd. What was it about my husband? I had not experienced any form of enlightenment during my marriage, and I was stuck on conventional medical concepts. Also, I knew nothing about past lives and karma. The whole experience remained a mystery to me until I realized that I developed cystitis only with my ex-husband.

Then one day I met Leonard Orr and I learned about Rebirthing/Breathwork. I became more conscious of the metaphysical causes of conditions, and I started getting serious about alternative healing. Once before a training session in Boston, I had a dream that five men came into my room and left a tarantula on the bed. I awoke, terrified and screaming. The next morning at the coffee shop, five men came in and sat down with me at my table! I panicked but tried to remain calm. During the sex therapy section of the training, I nearly fainted. Fortunately, my trainer continued with the session. I pulled out a piece of paper and did some automatic writing: "Five men, rape, Africa." After that, I found myself on the floor in a spontaneous Breathwork session.

Was my ex-husband one of those men? Some alternative healers have found that when we are younger, we often are attracted to past-life mates with whom we have karmic experiences that need to balance out. We must do this before we can move on to more loving and whole relationships. I realized my history of cystitis was related to my past life karma with my husband who had raped me before. The day after the session in Boston, I happened to have an appointment with a famous aura reader. She told me I had almost totally worked out that karma. Prior to that, I had never understood how past-life experiences could come back to inflict our current bodies. I healed from cystitis. It was a matter of bringing up the cause and letting it go!

Migrating Pain

In addition to insomnia after my father died, I began to experience a lot of physical pain in my body. This condition developed right after I saw my father in his casket. The pains were intense at times, and they migrated around my body. The whole experience was unusual for me, because prior to my father's dying, I hadn't had any pain. I realized that it must be all psychosomatic, and I knew that doctors could not help me. I learned to live with pain for fourteen years until I began Breathwork. After three sessions of Rebirthing, the mysterious pains left my body and never returned! It was a question of breathing out the "death urge" that had been taken in from my family and activated in me. Now you can understand why I became a Breathworker!

Hair Loss

My hair was always naturally curly. It had gotten so curly while I was in Florida that I bought straightener and almost ruined my hair. That was nothing compared to what happened to my hair after my divorce. It began falling out to the point that I had a large bald spot, and I wore a wig to hide it. The more

I worried, the more hair I lost. I was a nurse, so I had access to the best doctors. I went to so many that it became ridiculous, but none of them could help me. I was in constant therapy; that did not help either. I was desperate and really scared. This all happened prior to my first Breathwork experience and my metaphysical awakening. I was still deeply entrenched in the modern medical approach to healing. Nothing worked and I became nearly suicidal, which made it even worse.

One day in Phoenix, I visited yet one more dermatologist. I decided he would be the final one. I was fed up! He had white hair and was a sweet father figure. I trusted him. He suggested that I save the amount of hair that fell out each week and bring it to him. He wanted to determine if the loss increased or decreased. It always increased, and the bags of hair got fuller.

One week he looked at me and said, "My dear, you have a VERY serious problem."

"You're telling me!" I shrieked. "You are my last hope. I cannot stand to go to another doctor."

He went to his prescription pad wrote the following: "Read this book: *Peace of Mind* by Rabbi Lieberman."

I was shocked and wondered, "What kind of prescription is this?" I read the book and was blown away. It was my first real exposure to metaphysical philosophy. It explained how the mind rules the body. Why hadn't any of the nursing books I had studied covered this? I will always be grateful to that man. My hair stopped falling out, but I still had quite a bald spot. I was starting my third year of this condition.

I remember looking into the mirror and saying, "What if this never ends?" I dealt with this fear every day. After one year of Breathwork, I had worked out almost all the tension that prevented my hair from becoming healthy. I had some help at that time from my friend, Dr. Irv Katz. He did a couple of hypnotic sessions with me. I trusted him as he was a fellow Breathworker, LRT graduate (of my Loving Relationship Training which I had started to teach by then), sex therapist, and a great psychologist. He got me right down to all my unconscious issues of loss. Between the Breathwork and the sessions with Dr. Katz, I was healed. My hair grew back! It was a miracle for me, and my friends could not believe it. I went on a marvelous trip to Hawaii and was finally free of that condition. The whole experience was a powerful lesson for me.

The issues of loss from my childhood had manifested into a real, physical condition of loss in my body. My mind, conscious or unconscious, really did rule my body!

Food Neurosis

I was born on the kitchen table, so maybe my food neurosis started then. My birth trauma was all wired up with food. I was not breast fed and that was also a huge issue for me. In one of my past-life regression experiences, I learned I was a leader and had been poisoned by food. Maybe it all started then. I was always neurotic about food, even as a child. I was terrified of getting fat, and I ate like a bird. To gain even five pounds drove me insane. It was my own private and inner hell.

My mother was a home economics teacher, and we lived in the heart of the Midwest where much of the nation's food is grown. Everyone at home was obsessed with food—it seemed that way to me, anyway. In the morning, you get up, think about breakfast, prepare breakfast, eat breakfast, and then clean up after breakfast. Then you think about lunch, prepare lunch, eat lunch, and clean up after lunch. Then you think about dinner, prepare dinner, eat dinner, and clean up after dinner. You go through the whole cycle over and over having even a bedtime snack. My mother was always concerned with what to eat with what. The only disagreements we ever had were in the kitchen and were about what to cook or how to prepare it. And then there was my father who took twelve different pills at every single meal. He laid them all out on his plate, which reminded me of his illness and that he might be dying. I could not relax at meals. I wanted to get out of there and away from the obsession with food.

At one point in my life, I got so neurotic about eating that I began to fear eating off my own plate. This got especially intense when my past-life stuff was coming up. What if my food was poisoned? I became increasingly paranoid and had to eat off one of my friends' plates. Fortunately, most of my friends were understanding. They would tell me to take a walk around the block or something, which helped me get a grip on myself.

In the late seventies, my neurosis came to a head while visiting my guru Babaji in India. Once, in His presence, I became very nervous and obsessed with the subject of food. I was not overweight at all, but I constantly worried about it. I lived on the edge of anorexia all the time, but it was ridiculous for me to experience those fears in Babaji's ashram. I decided to confess my obsession to Him, for I was on the verge of severe neurosis. I could not even concentrate in the temple. One day I walked right up to Him and said, "Babaji, I am totally obsessed and neurotic about the topic of food."

He looked at me and abruptly said, "Oh, just give up food," and walked away.

I took this very seriously. Was He implying that I should become a breatharian and be like Saint Teresa Newman who ate only one communion wafer a day for twenty-five years? I went back to Babaji and asked him if He meant immediately.

"No, the food here is holy and blessed. You give up food when you go back to America."

I was still a neophyte around Babaji. I took everything that He said literally. I did not understand His ways, His methods, or His *lilas* (divine tricks or play by the master to help you crack your issues). What followed then was difficult. I was not a vegetarian at the time, and I began to have visions of sizzling steaks going right by me in the temple and in the presence of Babaji. Then I would see large pizzas, dripping with cheese. I had never had visions before; but these visions were in vivid color and kept getting stronger. I could no longer pray, chant, or meditate. I was losing my mind.

Finally, one evening I knelt before Babaji and once again told the truth: "I've gone crazy now." Suddenly, He picked up two large cymbals, the kind that one sees in a marching band. He raised them up over my head and crashed them together with such force that my body shook wildly. And then it was over. My mind cleared completely. Babaji had given me a type of "sound healing." Later I realized I had never seen those cymbals around Him before that moment, nor did I see them any time thereafter. Had He materialized a set of cymbals for my healing? Was it all a dream?

And yet, still taking Babaji literally, when I left India, I gave up food as He had told me to do. He had also told me to walk every morning at 4 o'clock. I was in Hawaii and gave up food for thirty days. Every morning I got up and walked. I was not hungry, but I felt angry. I took long walks to clear the anger. After thirty days of this routine, I realized it was all a lila, and the point of it was for me to process some of my anger about food and death. I started to feel better and eat normally.

There were a few setbacks, though. I was fine until some friends and I piled into a car and drove to Mexico for a lobster feast. We were on a beach with mariachis playing, and unlimited platters of lobster kept coming. I wondered how my friends could eat so much and still be so happy. I reached my limit right away, and then my fear came up again. On the way home from that trip, I curled up in the fetal position in the back seat and prayed to Babaji and Jesus for liberation. I pleaded once again for help. Then I heard the words *The only diet there is,* and I realized I was being told to write another book.

The Only Diet There Is was the hardest book I ever wrote. One-third of the way through, I got severe writer's block and could not write anything for a year. I was really struggling. But thanks to my friend R. R. who was a brilliant restaurateur, I broke through. He could eat any amount of food without gaining weight or getting full. He could eat seven-course meals over and over. I picked his brain and asked him to explain how he could do that. When he explained his mindset to me, I did not totally "get it" but whatever he said worked anyway. The next day I broke through my writer's block and food neurosis, and was able to finish the book, which I dedicated to him. "The Ego and Food" chapter put it all together. Afterward it did not matter what I ate, and I stopped thinking about the whole issue. I had always wanted to be able to eat anything and not gain weight. By the time I really achieved that, I was bored with food altogether. I was finally liberated. It felt like heaven to be free of that ridiculous pattern.

Arthritis

All my healing issues were beginning to dissolve as I came deeper into metaphysical understanding. I was beginning to feel good. It was a thrill to be at the beginning of Breathwork and studying with Leonard Orr. I was over my divorce, had a new boyfriend, and we were in San Francisco during the heyday of the alternative consciousness movement. We lived in a spiritual community, and Leonard Orr was teaching us the concepts of physical immortality. I had already been working out my unconscious death urges the hard way, so I adapted quickly to Leonard's ideas. I wanted to live, and I wanted to be healthy. I was ecstatic to learn that I may be able to prolong my life. I gave up nursing and modern medicine that year; one day I just walked out. Why should I stay in a profession that did not produce the quick and permanent healing I was seeing in rebirthing/Breathwork?

I was so enthusiastic about rebirthing that I told Leonard I thought I should write a book for Breathworkers and include the information on physical immortality. Most of that information was underground, and I was beginning to explore it. I felt that my second book should be called *Rebirthing in the New Age*. I wanted to write it with Leonard, and I told him that we needed a chapter on physical immortality. That night we tossed the I Ching to see if the world was ready for such a book. The I Ching came out with the following: "Yes, but you are on very thin ice." I told him I decided to write it anyway if he would help me.

I locked myself in seclusion and began the chapter on physical immortality. I had no idea how much would come up from my subconscious mind. I was in a bit over my head. It was still such a radical thing to discuss. A few days into it, my fingers locked up with gripping pain. I ran crying into Leonard's room.

"Leonard," I shouted, "I have arthritis!" I knew I could have a brilliant writing career, and I was barely getting started. Now it might all be over!

He looked at me calmly and said, "Oh, this is great!"

"What do you mean?" I screamed at him. "How can this be great?"

Then he said it was great because I was going through my old age early and that he did not have to worry about me anymore. He was not concerned at all. I began to relax. (Only an immortalist could have gotten me through that moment.) I began rebirthing feverishly for three weeks to process out the arthritis. It worked! Breathwork had healed me again.

The important thing I learned is that we need to be in the presence of enlightened friends who do not go into agreement with our negative conditions. If Leonard had gotten upset, I would have been sunk and most likely would have arthritis to this day. This is exactly how Jesus healed people. He never affirmed their egos; he only saw them healed. I went through several other early aging symptoms after that. I became hard of hearing. I also released that with Breathwork.

Leonard Orr once said, "It is better to go through that stuff when you are young and strong enough to really process it."

Sinusitis

I was in Bali with close associates and friends. It was my birthday, and we were all having a great time. That afternoon I developed a sudden sinus block without any warning. I had not been sick for a long time, and I thought it would just pass. It did not pass, and later I realized that it started at the exact time of my birth, 2:30 in the afternoon, August 24. It took me awhile to put the connection together. I continued to travel, and the condition kept getting worse, especially because I was flying in airplanes a lot. I went from healer to healer and worked on myself constantly. By then, I had learned how to clear my mind much better; but it did not work on my sinus infection. Nothing I did helped, nor were the healers I visited able to clear the problem. When it finally sunk in that the condition really started at the exact time of my birth, I called Dr. Bob Doughten, the only obstetrician in the United States who was also a rebirther-Breathworker. He had been rebirthing the teenagers he had delivered years before! That impressed me, and I was anxious to see him.

I flew to Portland, where he lived, and I suggested that he rebirth me on the kitchen floor since I was born in the kitchen. He was more than willing. It is great to have a good Breathworker, but it is the ultimate to have an obstetrician guide your session! I told him I thought I needed to review my whole birth one more time. I asked him to imagine pulling me out. He put his hand on my head while I breathed. Then he suddenly said, "Oh, I see you were pulled out wrong." (My doctor at my home birth was a general practitioner, not an obstetrician)

I felt pain around my nose and shouted, "I am damaged!" I re-experienced my sinus area being nearly crushed by the doctor who had delivered me.

During my birth, I had stopped the birth process myself, waiting for my father to come back into the kitchen. He had gone out to the porch to light a cigarette! That is when the doctor tried to pull me out, but I wanted to wait a little longer. I remembered the whole scenario then and there. As you can imagine, cigarettes bothered me my whole life.

Dr. Doughten sat me up, looked into my eyes, and said, "You know that you have the power to heal this yourself, but you are not doing it. You are setting your life up in such a way that you must go back to modern medicine so that you are forced to forgive doctors." (Brilliant, no?) I knew he was right, and I promised him I would go.

In Denver, I opened the phone book to professional specialists in ENT. I ran my finger down the page, and it stopped at Dr. Roy Jones. The only appointment I could get was 2:30 in the afternoon, the exact time of my birth! I walked into his office and almost fell over. He looked exactly like Dr. Moore, my obstetrician! I could not believe it. I thought that it all had to be a Babaji lila, and I told my assistant Wendy to help me surrender to this doctor totally. I told her I was not going to fight anything that he said.

When he came back with the X rays, he said, "These are opaque four. I cannot possibly let you leave here without a surgery! You must avoid flying, and you are very lucky that you don't have optic nerve damage. I just cannot believe you have been walking around with this condition."

So, there it was. Did I dare confess to him my arrogance, that I thought I would never need a doctor again and that I had no insurance? He was very kind and understanding when I told him the truth. He arranged it so I could go in as an outpatient and go home right after the surgery if Wendy promised to look after me.

The last thing I ever wanted to do was to go back to modern medicine, but I remembered what Dr. Bob Doughten had said, and I humbled myself. The whole ordeal turned into a very spiritual experience. The nurses had read my books believe it or not! They were like angels. The night before, the surgeon introduced me to the anesthesiologist, saying that they had an excellent relationship and had gone to school together. That helped me relax. The next morning when I was on the gurney in the waiting room to go in, a surgeon came out and called my name. He said that my surgery went very well!

I thought I was losing it for a moment and said, "Wait a minute, I have not even gone in yet!"

He seemed confused and ruffled. Was he channeling my name or the outcome of the as-yet-unperformed surgery? I took it as a message from Babaji that everything was going to be okay. I went into operating room relaxed. Later, they told me that while under anesthesia, I gave everyone in the room a lecture on how dolphins were programmed by Atlanteans!! They were so amazed that they called in other staff to listen. It must have been funny..

Later I visited a healer in Madrid who was very strong but said little. I told him nothing about my ordeal. He passed his hand over my sinus area and said only, "Karmic break." Then he saw that I had allowed myself to be experimented on with some type of lasers in ancient Atlantis—something to do with the uplifting of humanity. (I can imagine myself doing that.)

The whole experience of severe sinusitis taught me that many, if not all, of our physical conditions are absolutely linked to our past. Whether it be past lives, birth traumas, or childhood conditioning, our illnesses and physical problems are almost always rooted in some form of negative, unconscious memory that we can discover and release through Breathwork and other methods of alternative healing.

Hypothermia

I took time off from my own healing journey and went home to see my sister, who had a diagnosis of melanoma. Her aura was quite dark, and she was very angry. I spent hours with her while she vented her feelings. I tried to help her as much as I could. I gave her lists of people who have healed themselves of her type of cancer. She would not look at the lists nor did she want to hear about that. I hoped that she would ask for help, but she did not. She was not interested in alternative healers, and she had refused to read my books. I was a heretic in her eyes.

When I left her that last time, I began to experience intense cold and freezing chills throughout my body. Apparently, I was channeling as much of my family's death urge as I could stand, which triggered more of my own. I shook and shook and could not get warm, no matter what I did. The cold got so intense that when I walked into a room, the heat from the venting systems turned cold and the hot water in the taps turned to cold water. It happened several times, even in my friend Fred's room. He was a personal witness to this bizarre phenomenon.

I could not shake the chills. Even when I wore a warm fur coat at the airports, people walked up to me and told me I looked really cold! Finally, I decided that a trip to the hot springs in California was in order. By a small miracle, I attracted a polarity therapist who was able to teach me how to treat my condition. He told me to stay in the hot thermal water for as long as I could stand it and then go directly into cold water. I could not imagine plunging into cold water, but he said it would "set the heat" in my bones. I followed his instructions exactly and it worked. I was able to connect with Mother Nature and heal through another bout with the death urge.

Melanoma

About six months after my sister died, I was in New Delhi with my then boyfriend. He was a yogi who had spent about ten years in India. Before that, he had been a doctor. By the grace of Babaji, he was there with me. He happened to notice a mole on my left leg and told me it was serious and needed to be removed. I had not even noticed anything wrong; it looked like something ordinary to me. I was working hard to tune out illness and my past connections with ordinary medicine; to not dwell on them. However, I could tell he was channeling, and I figured I had better listen to him. When we returned to the U.S., I went to get it checked. Sure enough, it was melanoma. I was shocked; I was not the cancer type at all. Was I going into sympathy with my sister? Was it my last-ditch approach to win her love by being like her and manifesting the same death symptoms? As it was, the melanoma was not very deep, and they were able to get it all.

Exactly one year after my sister's death I was in Atlanta when, without warning, I threw myself on the bed while screaming, "I want to live! I want to live!" I called my friend Rhonda to help me. For four days, I went through intense paranoia about dying, and I did not want to be alone. There was nothing wrong with me physically whatsoever. Rhonda's son was there, and he had happened to cut himself and needed to see a doctor. I went with them and mentioned my fear condition to the doctor. When I told him it had been exactly one year since my sister died, he replied, "It is very common for family members to have strong reactions on the anniversary of a loved one's death." His words cleared me.

Later, in Bali again I woke from a horrible nightmare in which I saw my sister and she was deranged. She was driving the car and trying to kill me in it. I woke up screaming and saw that another spot of skin cancer on my leg had popped up overnight! It had not been there before that dream. I was confused and could not understand what was going on. I went to my altar and started praying. I was uncomfortable about seeing a doctor in Indonesia. My next stop on the trip was India, where I went to see a doctor who was a Babaji devotee. He looked up at the pictures of our guru and said, "Let's see what the old master has in store for you."

He called the chief surgeon of Delhi who had studied in London and was one of the best. I could handle that. The clinic was marginal, but I trusted him. He told me I needed to have it removed quickly. I was not going to mess around with melanoma! That form of cancer can move very fast, so I decided to go ahead with the surgery and process my mind later.

Fortunately, I was on my way to Rajasthan to see my guru Shastriji. I cried at his feet and begged him to explain what was going on with me. What he said to me then gave me the shock of my life.

He said, "I regret to tell you, but your sister has not crossed over properly. She has been entering your body to get your attention because she knows that you are the only one advanced enough to help her."

"What?" I asked. "How can this be?" These weird things could not possibly happen to *my* family. Was he talking about possession?

He told me I had to follow his instructions exactly, and that if it didn't work, I would have to go to Benares, the place where souls cross over. Benares —I could not believe it! Shastriji also told me I had to immediately chant five thousand mantras for her and perform a ceremony. I would have to perform this ceremony in the Ganges for the dead and wait to see if my sister would appear to me again. I did exactly what my guru instructed, but let me tell you, it was one of the hardest tasks in my life.

I had never tried five thousand mantras before. I did one thousand a day for five days. I focused almost all my attention on my sister. While in Delhi, I became terrified at the thought of not being able to complete what Shastriji had instructed me to do to help my sister. What if her soul stayed lost in the cosmos for thousands of years? I got really scared and was so upset that I went next door to the hotel room of my friends, Carmen and Adolfo. I got in bed with the whole family, and they held me while I worked on my breathing. Adolfo was my perfect Breathworker. He shared with me how his brother had died in his arms from an overdose of drugs.

My "group" that year in India consisted of students coming from all over the world and they were about to arrive at the hotel. I had to recover! I put my whole soul into that Breathwork session, finished my mantras, and all the fear cleared just five minutes before I was to meet my students. Later I performed the ceremonies just as Shastriji had instructed. My sister appeared to me, and she seemed all right. I obviously had something to work out and clear with her to stop manifesting cancer in my body. I went to a few past-life therapists and reviewed my karma with my sister. I received amazing information. If I had not worked through that and released it, I surely would have struggled with more bouts of melanoma. I recovered from the melanoma; however, for years I had other minor skin cancers on my legs. I did not permanently recover until I cleared my guilt about not having been able to heal my sister.

After that ordeal, I found peace with my issues about modern medicine. Often, people have fear about self-healing and must rely on doctors for help. Self-healing can be a deep and complicated issue, and we all need help to make the gradual transition to alternative healing methods. I have found that prayer helps and that through prayer, we can always attract the perfect healers when we need them.

Rheumatism

After my first experience of writing a chapter on physical immortality (when I got arthritis), I was terrified of the prospect of writing a whole book on the subject. It took me nine years to get up the courage. We did not have computers in those days. When I finally decided it was time to tackle this project, I bought a new electric typewriter. To my dismay, the typewriter kept blowing up, and I had to keep taking it back.

"Ma'am," the man at the store said, "you're too powerful. You must upgrade."

I had to keep upgrading typewriters until I finally had the most expensive model they had. But then the lights in my flat starts blowing out, and a lot of strange things began to happen in my apartment. I was busy writing, and I didn't let it bother me that much. It felt as though other forces were at work around me and coming through me. There was a force of resistance as well but, I got through it.

Shortly afterward, the book on physical immortality was released. I remember when I saw the first hardback edition: I was signing books in Los Angeles, and the line for autographs was longer than I had experienced. As the last people in line reached me, I felt a strange reaction. I felt old and heavy as lead, like I was aging rapidly.

The next morning, I was preparing to speak about physical immortality at a local Los Angeles church. While I was dressing, I experienced a sensation of shattering glass in my left hip, and I fell to the floor. The pain was terrible. I crawled to the phone and called a friend who was an excellent psychic. I pleaded with him to tell me what was happening. He said that the topic of my presentation was opposed to the teachings of the church and that I was meeting resistance. I told him I was going despite what was blocking me. I cried in the taxi all the way to the church while lying down in the backseat. I was having a spontaneous Breathwork session.

When I arrived at the church, I immediately told the staff I needed to lie down. "How much time do I have?" I asked.

"Twenty minutes. And the only place to lie down is in the kitchen," someone said. This was perfect, of course, because I had been born in a kitchen.

Some of the Breathworkers in the audience saw me coming in, realized I was in trouble, and got up to help me. I was crying and breathing like mad, trying to get ready for my talk, but the time ran out. Someone opened the swinging door and shouted, "You're on!"

My eye makeup was running, my Ungaro suit was wrinkled and getting spotted; I could hardly walk. My body felt like old age was setting in fast. It was clear to me that I had developed the symptoms of rheumatism. I had to be helped to the stage. I was a mess and hardly capable of lecturing on *How to Be Chic, Fabulous, and Live Forever!* I told the audience that I had to go through this in front of them. People started crying in the audience, and some of them went into spontaneous Breathwork sessions right there.

Suddenly, my energy shifted, and I delivered a lecture on the immortals of the Bible. I don't remember any of it except that I was given a standing ovation. After that, I was back on the kitchen floor in pain. At home, I stayed on a couch most of the afternoon, unable to move.

I remembered that two days before, someone had put the phone number of an acupuncturist in my coat pocket. I went for a treatment, and it helped me a lot. At least I was able to get on my feet and walk. But for the next few days, when I visited my Breathwork clients in Hollywood, I hobbled like someone who was old and decrepit. It was embarrassing. On top of that, I was scheduled to go to Australia. For three weeks, the severe symptoms of rheumatism persisted. I had chiropractic and all kinds of other treatments. When I got back to the home, I called my mother to ask her how she was.

"Oh", she said, "I had a real bad spell with my hip these past weeks but now it's gone." Later that day my hip suddenly healed, and I have not had the problem since. What was it with my family and me? Was my health that psychically connected to theirs? Was this their stuff or mine?

After that experience, I became confused about all my strange physical conditions and my sensitivity to other people's illness and death. I knew Babaji could process other people's stuff and worlds of karma through His body all the time, but He knew how to do it. I was obviously not very good at it. I began to wonder where the boundaries of my being were.

Gastritis and Anorexia

I was working in the Berlin shortly after the Wall came down. Everything was depleted in the atmosphere. I was sensitive to the personal and social trauma that surrounded it. My two nieces were in Germany, and my mother came to visit us. There we were, meeting together for the first time since my sister died. I had just learned that my niece had been pregnant when her mother (my sister) passed on. The baby was born with mild problems. We were all emotional wrecks, and it was too much for me. I could not digest it and I could not digest Berlin. Out of nowhere, I developed a terrible pain in my upper intestines. I could not eat, and I wondered if I had manifested an ulcer.

Like so many times before, I was privileged to have a wonderful assistant. This one was an obstetrician. She was amazing—also a trained Breathworker and a rock star! She was fun to be around and cheered me up.

For the first time in quite a while, I really had a chance to talk with my mother. I asked her if I had suffered with colic or something as an infant.

To my shock, she said, "Yes—for six weeks."

I asked why I had colic and she said, "Oh, some babies have colic, and some don't."

That answer did not satisfy me at all. I told her it had probably been caused by cow's milk and that I thought I was angry that she had not breast-fed me. She was understanding and agreed that maybe I was right. She explained that she could not breast feed me because she had developed a cyst breast feeding my sister.

Later I asked my assistant to give me a deep Breathwork session on the issue of breast-feeding. I went back to the time of my infancy and found that I had feelings and preverbal thoughts that translated to something like this: "I can never forgive this. I will never get over this. They might as well have put me out in the street!" I was angry that I had not been breast-fed. No wonder I had suffered with colic as an infant, and no wonder I had developed gastritis as an adult.

I started to pray very hard to Babaji. I cried at my altar and pleaded with Him to help me. I wondered how I was going to do a whole European tour when I could not even eat. Then a miracle happened. I was doing a seminar with mostly German people. An Italian man walked in late. I could not understand what he was doing there, and I wondered if he could understand German or the translation into English.

At the break, we ended up in the same elevator, and he introduced himself as Michelangelo. I suddenly blurted out, "Oh, you are the one from Italy. Please come to my room after we finish." I was startled at myself for being so direct. The words just came out of my mouth, but I had learned before to trust these things. He seemed to have no problem with it at all. (He later became my organizer in Italy.)

He came to my room later. He was a divine being, an angel. To my amazement, he told me he was a devotee of Babaji and Muniraj like myself! He said he had been *called* to come, that he had been in a car wreck on the way, but felt he still had to make it to the seminar. It was another Babaji miracle for me. I felt compelled to tell him about my condition, and he said he could help. He pulled some very fine, high-vibration food out of his bag. It looked like vegetable pâté and baby food. He fed me as if I were an infant, and I was able to eat a little. My prayers had been answered.

He told me he could heal me in two weeks if I could travel to Milan. It was a nice idea, but I had a scheduled tour to complete and could not arrange to get away. During the rest of the trip, I ate a teaspoon of bee pollen each day and a few fresh dates. I was unable to eat anything else, literally. It seemed like I had acute anorexia now.

During this period, people began telling me I needed to take time off, which was the last thing I wanted to hear. I was a workaholic who could not stop. But then, perfect strangers started walking up to me on the street and telling me I needed to take time off! This happened so many times that I realized Babaji must be speaking to me through other people, and I had better wake up.

I canceled part of my tour and rented a cottage on Cape Cod. Then I sent Michelangelo a plane ticket as he had agreed to come and stay with me for a few weeks. The day before he came, I decided to ask him to shave my head. I was in trouble with my body, and I wanted to facilitate the maximum healing possible. I prepared an altar in my cottage. Then I fixed a basket with all the necessities for the head shaving (mundan). I covered the basket with a sacred cloth and put it under the altar. I even called an astrologer to ask when the best time would be. She was astonished that I had chosen the Fourth of July. It was perfect, and she suggested one minute before midnight.

That night one of my students picked up Michelangelo at the airport and drove him to my cottage. It was good to see him. I immediately reminded him of my desire to have my head shaved, and he was agreeable. He had no problem accepting the sacred responsibility. He had his head shaved several times and he understood the deep meaning and power of this type of healing. We both had the same guru after all!

We started the mundan one minute before midnight. It took quite a while and I was awake all night. I had shaved my head twice before, and I thought a third time would be a snap. But I was shocked at how spiritually strong it was. I lay on the couch for days feeling my chakras swirling, and I felt as though I were turning inside out.

Michelangelo began giving me hour-and-a-half sessions of reflexology twice a day. He is a master, and his touch was very intense. He also prepared and fed me his high-vibration pate each day. It was hard for me to digest even small amounts, but I managed them. After about ten days, I began a healing crisis and started to go kind of berserk. He helped me by taking me for long walks and making me walk faster and faster, which got my breathing into a constant Breathwork mode. The final week he took some time to go to one of my Loving Relationships Training (taught by co-trainers) in Connecticut. It was my gift to him. When he came back, he was excited but had gone through an energy shift himself. He ended up on the floor, breathing through his own healing crisis before he went back to Italy! He said the training was like a steam roller for him.

By the end of his visit, I was much better. I left Cape Cod and went to Bali for a rest. It was wonderful to be on that island and with a shaved head! I was so glad I had taken some time for self-healing, and I was so grateful to Michelangelo.

After Bali, I went to India. I wanted to give my thanks and prayers to Babaji. While I was in the Himalayas, I met a beautiful Dutch man. We really hit it off and both felt we had been together in a past life as young lovers in Poland. Well, it just so happened that I was scheduled to do the first LRT ever given in Poland right after my mission in India. Naturally, my new friend decided to travel with me.

The whole experience of gastritis taught me that an adult healing crisis often directly relates to a childhood or infancy crisis. In my case, I was able to bring up my feelings of lack and anger at not being breast-fed and deal with them. I was able to let them go and to get healing before they ate a hole in my body. I was eternally grateful that I was able to expand my awareness beyond modern medicine and traditional religion.

P.S. The reason it took me so long to get over those conditions is because back then I had no idea that
I had a subconscious thought, "I might not get over this." One has to handle doubt. If I can get over all of the above, so can you get over anything.

My Latest Healing

After marrying Markus, I felt quite healthy *until* the 2020 Pandemic and the Great Sequester hit. The very day that it was announced as such on the news I started having diarrhea. I thought it must be due to the fear in the world and my own fears. However, processing that did not seem to help and it continued and continued. At one point I panicked and I went the medical route, and even had a colonoscopy (which turned out normal). I took several rounds of parasite treatments as I had traveled in many third world countries previously. Nothing helped. I consulted medical mediums who gave up on me. I even had black stools at times, which I figured out was due to the unconscious death urge. Fortunately, by understanding *that,* I did not panic more. I prayed a lot.

Finally, toward the end of the pandemic we were able to go back to Babaji's ashram in India and a healer there named Gloria helped me to see a past life that I was not previously willing to see. It was too awful. I was a healer in Iraq and there was a very, very serious pandemic. Of course, there were no vaccinations back then and everyone was dying. In fact, they were starving and dying of starvation and I felt helpless. I got better after that but I was still not perfect. Even though I was figuring out the consciousness factors, I did not realize that I had an unconscious thought, "I might never get over this." That thought hindered my healing. When I realized that, I worked a lot on *Faith.*

I kept praying and what finally worked was the following formula, the list of things that really helped me get over my conditions:

- ❖ Faith
- ❖ Some Homeopathy
- ❖ Lords of Karma prayers from Diane Stein's work
- ❖ Past life Regressions with Gloria
- ❖ Re-writing *Healing and Holiness*
- ❖ Creating the *Revolutionary Spiritual Healing Seminar*

❖ Private Liberation Breathing sessions
❖ A lot of processing my thoughts with Markus
❖ *Mantra Breathing*® (a new thing we are doing in the sessions when we breathe to a mantra being sung or recited)
❖ Finishing my newest book: *Outside the Box with Babaji*
❖ Getting back to traveling and doing our work on the road.

I am very happy to say that the above formula finally worked!! One reason it took me so long to get over THAT was because I was not taking into consideration it might be a past life. Babaji finally got through to me on that by directly sending me Gloria Otero, the past life reader/healer who came with us on the India Quest 2022 to Herakhan.

> **By the way, my guru Babaji always told us, "Faith is everything!" Start with that! And give up the thought, "I'll never get over this!"**

2.

The Basics of Metaphysical Healing

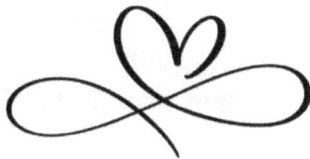

Note: Some things in this book are repeated a few times. That is deliberate. People remember things better when repeated.

Jesus says in A Course in Miracles that the Holy Spirit will free us from sickness, death, pain and suffering. That is why we need to turn over our thoughts that cause these conditions to the Holy Spirit. There is a Higher Power in us that we can tap into, and we must make direct contact with this Power of Love if we are to heal ourselves. But first we have to understand how we brought about the sickness in the first place.

Causes of Sickness and Pain

❖ The mind rules the body. All illness is *mental illness.* All physical conditions are triggered by pre-existing sub-conscious thoughts.

- The body is at the effect of the mind.
- Negative thoughts produce negative results in the body.
- All sickness comes from the belief in separation from *God,* or the *Source of Life,* if you'd rather call It that.
- The sick remain *accusers.* They cannot forgive.
- In sickness, we are punishing ourselves rather than have God punish us for our "guilt."
- Any time we are sick, we are replacing God with the ego (fear, anger, guilt, isolation, etc.)
- All forms of sickness are physical expressions of fear.
- If you are sick, you are withdrawing from The Christ's Healing Energy/God and yourself.
- All pain and symptoms are the effort involved in clinging to a negative thought.
- Chronic pain and illness are caused by repressed anger and rage.
- Sickness is competition with God.
- Cancer is a battle between the life urge and the death urge.
- The source of cancer comes from hopelessness and the desire to die.
- As long as you think "death is inevitable," you will create a sickness to prove you are right.
- Guilt demands punishment and makes you suffer with pain and sickness.
- Fighting with the condition in your mind strengthens the problem.
- Keeping a deep dark secret in your life is bad for your health.

❖ The degree to which you are not healthy has to do with the degree to which you are in resistance to that.

Principles of Healing

❖ You have 100% control over your mind but you must be willing to give up the position of *being a victim.*

❖ Anything can be cured. You create illness with your mind, and you can *uncreate* it with your mind.

❖ You will give up pain or the symptom when you see no more value in it.

❖ The real physician is the mind of the patient himself. The outcome of healing is what the mind of the patient decides.

❖ The health of the body is governed by the subconscious mind.

❖ The physical body will do what your mind believes.

❖ All things are possible. Gratitude can create miracles.

❖ See yourself with the ideal state and act as if you already have it.

❖ All healing is essentially the release from fear.

❖ All healing involves replacing fear with love.

❖ With innocence you can ward off any disease.

❖ All healing is the result of some kind of forgiveness. All forgiveness leads to healing.

❖ As you become willing to accept the help of God by asking for it, you will get it. Nothing will be denied your simple request (unless you sabotage it by doubting it).

- Ask the Holy Spirit to teach you the right perception of the body. The Holy Spirit is the invisible Power of the Life Force Itself.
- Healing that is of the Holy Spirit always works. Unless the healer always heals by Him, the results will vary.
- Anything you have created, you can uncreate.
- For healing to happen, the cells must receive and retain more light, and be released from the past restrictions, limitations, and imperfections. (That is why you need a technique like Liberation Breathing to help you release these restrictions and take in the light.)
- Most people say: "I won't be happy until I am healthy." But you will be healthy when you are happy! (Unhappiness is due to loss of connection with the Source.)
- Maharishi Mahesh Yogi said: "Bliss is the most powerful agent of physiology." (Joyful people are also healthy people.)
- There is a healing force within us—a kind of Divine Physician. (You know this because when you cut your finger it heals quickly.) This force is an intelligence that drives the immune system. Trust that.
- The Atonement heals with certainty. Say this: "I am one with God and I allow the Holy Spirit to undo all my wrong thinking."
- Infinite Love and Gratitude have the potential to affect the highest of frequencies which can harmonize the body.
- Healing begins when you love yourself unconditionally.

- ❖ The first step in healing is to be without judgment.
- ❖ It is in deep relaxation that the body heals most efficiently.
- ❖ Peace of mind is connected to physical health.
- ❖ Looking on the illness as an OPPORTUNITY to grow in self-awareness activates the potential for healing.
- ❖ Desiring to heal is not the same as having the WILL to heal. Some people who want to be healed don't have the will to make the life changes required. Strengthen your WILL.
- ❖ Healing can be understood as the natural consequences of nurturing a spiritual consciousness.
- ❖ To give a problem over to the Holy Spirit to solve for you means that you want it solved. To keep it for yourself to solve without His Help is to decide it should remain unsolved. The Holy Spirit's problem solving is the way the problem ends.
- ❖ The guiltless mind cannot suffer. If the unconscious guilt in the mind is healed, pain will not be felt.
- ❖ You must eliminate all doubt. You must re-own your power.
- ❖ With God (the Divine Life Force) all things are possible.
- ❖ There is no disease too small or too big for God (Deuteronomy 7:15 "And the LORD will take away from thee all sickness.") That is a promise.

It is so important to understand *the real physician is the mind of the patient himself.* The outcome of healing is what the mind of the patient decides. And God's Healing is already in your mind to access.

> *"You have healing power within you. Permanent Healing comes from freeing the mind which is in every cell of your body. Every cell is enveloped in thought. Your body is composed of radiant substance. The body is soft, pliable, and even plastic to your thoughts."* (Catherine Ponder: *The Dynamic Laws of Healing)*

If you do not want to believe that it is the mind that is the cause of the disease, you must be at least willing to consider that. You must have an open mind because otherwise you will remain a victim and will not learn to heal yourself.

Perhaps it will help to hear what Jesus says on the subject in Lesson #152 of A Course in Miracles, "The power of decision is my own."

> *No one can suffer loss unless it be his own decision. No one suffers pain except his choice elects this state for him. No one can grieve nor fear nor think him sick unless these are the outcomes he wants. And no one dies without his own consent. Nothing occurs but represents your wish.*

The text of ACIM also says that ALL disease is the wish to die and overcome the Christ. What is meant by the Christ in this statement is Being in a perfect state of health and happiness all of the time.

There is nothing that is incurable except that which you acknowledge as incurable. To change your body, all that you have to do is change your mind and your body will change automatically. This change of mind has to be total, though, free of doubt and fear.

> *The only thing that is required for a healing is a lack of fear. The fearful are not healed and cannot heal. Come to the Holy Instant and be healed. (ACIM Chapter 27; V.)*

LIBERATION BREATHING® is the most powerful way to heal yourself of past fears, anger, traumas, memories of problems and despair. We will discuss it in depth in Chapter 22. Our forms of Breathwork includes MANTRA BREATHING® as well, in which we breathe the circular, deep connected breath to the sound of powerful Sanskrit Mantras. (See the last chapter in which we discuss this.)

3.

Negative Thoughts and Personal Lies

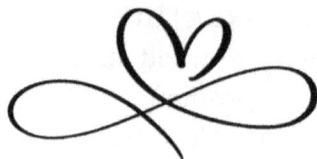

Personal lies can make you sick and keep you from healing yourself. In my other books, I often discuss how our most negative thoughts can affect our lives. These include negative, preverbal thoughts from birth and infancy. In this chapter, I try to show how these negative thoughts can sabotage our ability to heal ourselves. The *personal lies* are our most negative thoughts about ourselves, usually formed at birth, in the womb, or brought in as a core belief from a past life. Because they are not the *real* truth about us, we call them personal lies. Everyone has one. Until you find out what yours is, you cannot straighten out your life. Here are some of the most common personal lies we have seen in Liberation Breathing:

* ❖ I am wrong.
* ❖ I am bad.
* ❖ I am not good enough.

- ❖ I am not perfect.

- ❖ I am weak.

- ❖ I am guilty.

- ❖ I can't.

- ❖ I can't make it.

- ❖ I am a failure.

- ❖ Something's wrong with me.

- ❖ I am a disappointment.

- ❖ I shouldn't be here.

- ❖ I am unwanted.

- ❖ I am evil.

- ❖ I am stuck.

- ❖ I am nothing.

As a Liberation Breathing Practitioner, I made a point of keeping records of clients' personal lies. I came up with around 365 of them before I stopped counting. Then when Markus came into my life, we wrote a book on the subject called *Liberation: Freedom from Your Biggest Block to Pure Joy* (bit.ly/LibRay). People who have read this short book say it completely changed their life! There are three ways the personal lie affects a person.

1. The person's tendency is to act out the negative thought.
2. The person may be able to suppress it and overcompensate for it.
3. The person may project it onto someone else.

#1 For example, people whose lie is "I am bad" may act bad and do things that are bad, bringing upon themselves bad judgment from others and reinforcing the thought of badness in themselves.

#2 Or they may work very hard to keep the thought of being bad completely hidden from other people and overcompensate by acting especially good all the time. They may become obsessed with being good, not seeing that their behavior is only a cover-up. The thought *I am bad* is merely covered up. It becomes a booster for acting "really good." But underneath all their good achievements is the nagging feeling of something really bad.

#3 Or, finally, they may project their bad thoughts onto others and start seeing everyone else as bad instead of facing such defects in themselves.

These *personal lies* are like addictions. A person believes the thought so strongly that after years and years of accepting it, the thought seems normal. It also feels as though one's life almost totally depends on keeping that thought alive. The person starts believing that is who he or she really is. Having survived both birth and infancy with that thought, the person suffers an unconscious fear that he or she will die if they give up the thought. Of course, this does not make sense. It is totally insane. The opposite is the truth. Keeping the personal lie will kill you in the end. This is a destructive trick of the ego, because the ego secretly wants you *dead*.

Some people mistakenly think that as soon as they discover their personal lie, they can drop it overnight. However, people usually have a fear of an overnight shift in habit patterns. They fear too much light or too much of an energy change all at once. Most people tend to chip away at negative thoughts and let them go slowly over time.

These negative thoughts are in the deep subconscious, so most people might not even be aware they have a block unless they experience Breathwork or some similar purification technique. And when they discover the personal lie, they too often go into denial that this thought is running things in their subconscious. The following are examples of how some of these personal lies can interfere with healing.

I am not good enough: These people might accept the idea that they are not good enough to be healed. So, no matter how many healing opportunities have been given them, none will help, because deep down they believe they are not good enough to deserve the result of healing. So, they will create a *sabotage* pattern.

I am wrong: People who think they are wrong also think they deserve punishment, and illness may be the very punishment they think they deserve. These people may also attract the *wrong* diagnosis, the *wrong* medicine, the *wrong* doctor or healer, and they never get anywhere. They may even get stuck on working in the wrong part of their mind on the wrong issues.

I am not perfect: These people often make up little things wrong with their bodies so they can feel imperfect. They might be obsessed with the imperfections they create. As soon as they heal one imperfection, they make up another so they can make sure they are never perfect. Often, they are never satisfied with the doctor or healer they choose, and then project that the doctor or healer is imperfect. Even if they should find the perfect doctor or healer, they might set up their treatment to turn out imperfect so something goes wrong so they can remain imperfect.

I am weak: These people may make up an illness that results in a feeling of weakness. Then they can physically experience the fact that they are weak, thus manifesting the proof that they are weak. They might create an illness such as anemia, for example, or Epstein-Barr virus, chronic fatigue syndrome, or something else that saps their energy. Often, these people are premature at birth and get stuck in the thought "I am too weak to heal myself."

I am guilty: Because guilt demands punishment, this person makes sure he or she is punished somehow. They might become sexually promiscuous so they can continue the guilt cycle and come up with a sexually transmitted disease. They may create something such as herpes out of healthy, normal sex. They may punish themselves in numerous ways such as losing money, friends, or a good job to anything else that feeds the guilt and causes them to suffer. Of course, the most natural way to take out guilt is on the body, and these people may create not getting healed because they feel too guilty to deserve healing. The guilt itself causes their condition and at the same time it keeps them from healing the condition!

I can't, or I can't make it: Sometimes these people create mysterious illnesses or diseases that cannot be diagnosed. They think they absolutely can't be healed.

Thoughts of helplessness and despair get stretched out to "I can't let go ... I can't get rid of this ... I can't control my body." These people can really get stuck in the thought, "I can't let go of the thought I can't." (Not to worry, a trained Liberation Breathworker knows how to handle these conditions.)

I am a failure: Imagine a person trying to heal himself or herself with the unconscious thought, "I am a failure." It won't work! They have set themselves up to fail at self-healing before they even try. Failing repeatedly with the same healing techniques is a typical pattern that this person would manifest to prove the thought, "I am a failure." They may even set it up even for medicine to fail. This pattern brings up the death urge, and their condition will get worse fast.

Something is wrong with me: This personal lie is a sure bet that something wrong will be created in the body. For example, I have known women with fertility problems that had the "something is wrong with me" syndrome. They went from doctor to doctor trying to get proof of infertility. It drove them nuts if the doctors found nothing wrong. What they did not see was that the infertility problem was a result of this thought when nothing was really wrong at all. I have known women with fertility problems who gave themselves up as hopeless; yet, after they had Liberation Breathwork and had breathed out that thought, they became pregnant!

I shouldn't be here: This personal lie can be deadly because these people have such a strong death urge that they may go around creating near-fatal accidents and illness. They often live on the edge of personal disaster and brag to others about how many "near misses" with death they have had. Some who believe they shouldn't be here have a lot of out-of-body experiences and might be great clairvoyants. However, when they get sick, it can be hard for the doctors trying to keep them alive on this plane.

I am unwanted: People with this thought pattern are often attracted to people of the opposite sex who are not attracted to them so they can feel unwanted. The sadness of constant rejection can make them feel devastated and sick. The problem is compounded because often they cannot ask for the support they need to be healed because they believe other people do not want to help them since they are unwanted.

I am evil: This is a core belief usually brought in from a past life or several past lives. People of this type are very hard on themselves and believe they deserve severe punishment. They might unconsciously destroy everything good in their lives—business, relationships, and even their bodies. They cannot imagine that they deserve happiness and success or healing. These people need a lot of spiritual help. Some women who are former prostitutes have this thought. Even though they may not be prostitutes in this life, they manifest attributes of one who makes others believe they are as evil as they believe themselves to be. It is common for them to create incurable diseases to keep others away, feeling that they deserve no healing whatsoever.

I am stuck: These people may have been stuck in the birth canal. Later they get stuck in all kinds of situations or stuck with an ongoing weight problem.

Their minds may go in vicious circles trying to figure out how to change, but they often get nowhere because they get stuck. Pains and conditions get stuck in their bodies also.

I am nothing: These people have very low self-esteem; they may think they deserve nothing. Often, they manifest anorexia or other diseases that waste away the body. The sad part is that they almost never reach out for help, for they truly believe that nothing or no one exists out there to help them. They may turn atheistic and deny the love and support of God and the universe, believing instead that they are nothing and nothing can help them.

Although these negative thought patterns seem extreme, the truth is they are more common than most people realize, and Breathworkers see them daily. For decades, I have watched people wrestle with these deep-rooted thoughts and their effects. Liberation Breathworkers have gone through their own Breathwork, discovered their own personal lies, and have survived and overcome them. On the other side of these thoughts is a whole new life.

We hear often of the death of someone who had been a happy, healthy, and positive person. She or he may not even have been very old. People may say, "I just cannot understand why one so healthy died, loving life so much." Even people who appear happy and healthy may have deep-rooted negative thought patterns carried from birth or past lives that silently and unconsciously keep them from being able to live.

You could be one of the best healers in the world (and if you are, I salute you and hope to meet you someday) but all your work with a client can go down the drain if the person goes back to his or her addictions and personal lies. For your work to have more lasting or permanent effects, please consider suggesting Liberation Breathing to your clients. They will appreciate you the more, and your healing service will be more valuable in the end. Please also consider Liberation Breathing for yourself. Your own healing abilities will greatly improve after you discover your own birth and past life thought patterns. If you get good results now, imagine what you might get after eliminating your own personal lies.

A well-trained Liberation Breathworker will go after the personal lies in the first session with a client.

The Personal Lie Undo—Redo Process

Once you have identified yours, you can apply this set of thoughts to overcoming it. We call this "The Personal Lie Undo—Redo Process." Here is an example of this process, using the personal lie, "I am bad."

1. I forgive myself for thinking, "I am bad."
2. God did not create me "bad."
3. God created me only good.
4. I am as God created me.
5. Therefore, the thought "I am bad" is a lie.
6. I let go of my stubborn refusal to release that thought.
7. I ask the Holy Spirit to help me release that thought.
8. I am now willing to see myself as only good.

We highly recommend you read our book on this subject of the personal lie. One reason is that it lists over 365 personal lies, so you can look down the list and see which ones resonate with you. The book is *Liberation: Freedom from Your Biggest Block to Pure Joy,* and you can purchase it on Amazon.

You have to identify the right personal lie for you. It is very important that you work with the exact personal lie. The ego wants to distract you into thinking you have handled it, when in fact maybe you are working on the wrong one! That is why you need someone skilled in this work to help you identify it and uncover how it has been operating in your life over a long period of time.

4.

Family Loyalty

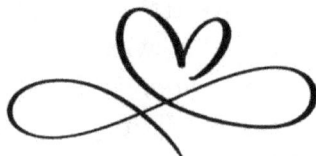

We may think we don't want to copy our parents, especially their *ailments,* but we feel a deep loyalty to our parents even if we do not feel close to them. In Breathwork, we have seen family loyalty take an unconscious form of copying not only parental behavior problems but also of copying parental illness and death patterns. It is an unconscious process and an unhealthy form of loving. People that are natural conformists manifest these patterns frequently. Rebels, on the other hand, are less likely to take on negative family patterns. Everyone, however, is susceptible to family loyalty to some degree.

When it comes to disease, many people say they inherited their disease. They may believe their disease is genetic and there is nothing they can do about it. But what if we could acknowledge the fact that we *choose* to go into agreement with our parents and the genes of our parents? What if we could change our genes and that parental agreement *with our minds*? One may think this is preposterous, but I know of cases where it has been done!

I once went out with a lawyer from Texas whose family had Huntington's Chorea. By all odds, he was supposed to have it too. It is a horrible disease of dementia. He said he had a 100% chance of getting it, and then he told me about the way he *chose* not to go into agreement with that disease. It was such a powerful experience for him that he could perfectly remember the day and time of his decision. He was only 12 at the time. He could remember everything that was in the room—the color and design of the carpet, curtains etc.—he saw everything exactly as it was at the time. To this day, his family doctors are mystified by his case and can't understand how he beat the odds. He is one who proved we do not have to inherit disease.

Shouldn't this story say something about what we tell our children? If we pass on our negative thoughts to them, they surely will have to struggle to overcome the potential illness, failure, and unhappiness these thoughts tend to manifest. How do we know when it is too late to change our genes? Is it ever too late? Miracle healing happens all the time and all over the world. I strongly recommend that you read *Quantum Healing* by Dr. Deepak Chopra if you still have doubts about the power of the mind to change the body.

Many people have already unconsciously programmed their own death to match that of a parent, grandparent, or loved one. This perpetuates the notion that one cannot do anything about inherited diseases. The statistics of such diseases then climb higher and that perpetuates the programming even more.

In my Physical Immortality seminars, I ask people to write down at what age they think they will die and of what condition. Their answers usually come out quite easily because their decisions were already made when they were children. When I ask them why they hold that belief about their death, they often reply that it is because of their first funeral experience or the death of a grandparent or loved one. The conditioning thought was "I guess I will be like him or her." A person can identify with a parent or a grandparent so strongly that they take on the body type, thought processes, and all.

A person's genetics can change! I have learned that a person's palm can reveal their genetics. One of my gurus was also a palmist. He read my palm once every seven years or so because the genetics information changes, according to him. Once I met a man in Russia who had no line at all on his palm. There was just a little X in the middle. I freaked out and asked what it meant. "Total mutation," he said.

Once in a healing seminar I was presenting, I had an idea for a new healing process: I had two people sit across from each other and record on paper all the symptoms and diseases that their mothers had, which of those they had copied, and why they had copied them. Then I had them do the same for their fathers and then for their grandparents. It was a lengthy process that grew so intense that I decided never to do it again unless an immediate Breathwork session took place afterward. I found myself personally doing the new process for weeks after that seminar. I processed out all disease programming that my grandmother had manifested in her body. Had I not been able to do Breathwork each step of the way, I am sure I would have ended up in big trouble. Frequently in my life, I had manifested premature aging and reversed it. I hope you will read our book *Physical Immortality: How to Overcome Death.*

The first step to mastering a pattern of excessive family loyalty is to recognize your tendency to copy. If you start getting a disease like that of one of your parents, grandparents, or ancestors, you do not have to resign yourself to it. Resignation can be deadly. It is possible to rise above the negative thought patterns. You may need the support of knowledgeable and advanced healers who know how to transform the mind and move energy.

The point is that *you can still love your parents without being loyal to all their negative patterns!*

In my case, I was a rebel, while my sister was a conformist. (She died at the same age my father was when he died.) A strange thing happened to me after she died. I unconsciously began to switch to being conformist, perhaps to get close to her or something. It felt very strange and did not work for me at all. The whole experience threw me into confusion for a while, and I did not know who I really was. I started to lose my grip. I started to take on my sister's mind, her disease, and whatnot. I also felt guilty that I lived, and she did not, and I made up ways to suffer for this guilt. It took me nearly five years to straighten myself out and let those patterns go. It was all an unconscious process, and I found it was amazing as I watched it all play out.

Never underestimate the power of the subconscious mind and the ego's trickery. Why do you suppose the masters strongly recommend that we stay on the spiritual path? We must be alert, for one thing. And we must learn techniques to handle all the unconscious stuff.

I am not a geneticist and I do not want to get into arguments with geneticists. What I want to point out is this: if someone can materialize his body and dematerialize his body at will, as I have witnessed my guru Babaji do, then there is a lot about the human mind we don't understand!

If you still think all this is crazy, try reading books written about the ancient teaching of the masters in India. I strongly recommend the series by Robert E. Svoboda titled *Aghora: At the Left Hand of God* and *Aghora II: Kundalini.* It is incredible material, and I can hardly digest it. What these writings have taught me is that there is something far beyond what we currently call modern science. There is the Divine Mother—the Eternal One who is Supreme and the Great Healer. If you are stuck in a family disease, start praying to the Divine Mother.

5.

Addiction to Suffering

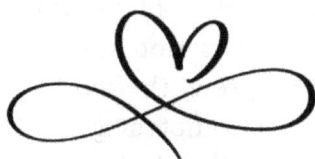

It took a long time to notice that I had such an insidious addiction to suffering because when compared to most people, I seemed okay. Yes, I had gone through devastating experiences and had endured many unhealthy conditions in my body, but at least I was not in and out of hospitals, and so on. I felt quite resilient; pleased that I had not become bitter from the trials of life. I was not depressed or moody. Most of the time I was happy despite my symptoms and felt fortunate to travel about freely. Even though I was not uber rich, I had more than enough money. My symptoms were not counted as a form of suffering, I just blamed them on overwork. However, this mistake kept me from facing the area of my mind that I needed to face.

When I got serious about healing *all* my symptoms, I had to do an in-depth study of myself to learn why I was not letting them go. I discovered that because of my religious upbringing, I thought I needed to suffer in some way because the church said suffering is "holy." If I wanted to be holy, and I did, then I could never have the perfect life free of suffering. "If you suffer now, you get to heaven later," I was taught. So, there it was—always making sure I had some symptoms. I would heal one and accept another. That way I could be sure I was not perfect and that I was suffering.

As I grew enlightened and happier, it seemed I should suffer *more* because of the guilt of being too happy. (In church, one is not supposed to be TOO happy.) The happier I grew, the worse my symptoms became, so that I could not stay happy. That was insane! I started resenting the church again which was a dangerous attitude according to church warnings. If you dare question the church, you will surely suffer, and even more later. You may "go to hell."

Oh, I was able to function all right. I was able to work and even have a fairly good time—but something always kept me from experiencing ecstasy. It seemed to elude me. And that something turned out to be my ego, of course, mainly the part of my ego that was trying to convince me that I had to suffer.

After I recognized this pattern and started to give it up, my mind went into the next phase: a new reason to suffer. Others are suffering. I should be like others if I am to be here and want to be close to them. After all, I could not be the only one around in perfect health! I would be too different. And I was already too different. People might think I was a fake. I had better suffer somewhat to be accepted, to be considered "normal." This was the next trick of my ego.

On top of this nonsense, somehow, I had it wired up that if I had symptoms like my father and sister, both of whom had died, I would somehow still be connected to them. If I became totally healed, I might want to stay here and then I might not get to go to "heaven" and be with them again. Furthermore, I felt guilty that I was able to live, and that guilt made more symptoms. All this was unconscious, mind you. It is a wonder I did not land up in the hospital. I had to stay on top of it constantly for that not to happen. It was a lot of work to keep ahead of this guilt I inherited from my religious upbringing. Fortunately, I had read A Course in Miracles, which says, "God's will for us is perfect happiness." This book, this correction of religion, helped me straighten out this mess.

Then one day in India while visiting the great saint, Shastriji, I noticed that he was always in ecstasy. He kept shouting to me, "I want you to have intense joy!" Now, try to imagine the effect that had on me. There he was—the living example of what I wanted to be! That is what I needed to see, what I needed to hear. And it was *real*. That is why I went to India in the first place: I needed examples. In one's spiritual life, such experience is called "The Principle of Right Association." You associate with that which you want to become. You hang out with those who force you to *adapt upward*.

I recommend that you become aware of all the forms of suffering you might be creating. One can create suffering in the body, at work, in a relationship, even on vacation. Become committed to giving up suffering. Talk to Jesus about it, to Babaji, to the Divine Mother. Pray about it. This process should also help you become aware of all that you feel guilty about.

Read A Course in Miracles until you unravel all false religious theology. There *is* a way out. Keep studying it until you absolutely know that you are innocent, and that guilt is not of God. For meditation and affirmative prayer, employ A Course in Miracles lessons: "God's will for me is perfect happiness." "I choose the joy of God instead of pain." "Other people's suffering is not my own." "I can be free of suffering today." "God in His mercy wills that I be saved from suffering."

Suffering is a pattern. It can be an addiction. We may think we need to suffer to be holy. This is false religious theology. One has to say, "I give up my addiction to suffering to the Holy Spirit."

We must forgive the church for teaching us that suffering is holy. We have had that programming for lifetimes. Are we ready to let go of church dogma and not feel guilty about it?

One can give up their suffering to Shiva. Shiva is the part of God that destroys ignorance. When we say we are giving something up to Shiva, we are saying that we really don't want it anymore. We must have real conviction to give it up!

Addiction to suffering is one of the reasons that prayers for healing do not work. We could have the exact right prayer but if we are still addicted to suffering, we will unconsciously keep the problem so we can suffer.

We tend to think about things that are bothering us instead of good things. It is an addiction to focus on what is bothering us. If one is suffering from a condition, it is important to ask and answer, "What am I punishing myself for by having this condition?"

One must get in touch with the part of the mind that does NOT want things to work. When we are sick and suffering, we have lowered our frequency and then we become susceptible to bad things.

The reason it was so hard for me to give up suffering is because I felt disloyal to the church and to my family if I were to give it up. Disloyalty was bad in my mind. What finally worked for me was to understand that I could choose to be loyal to Jesus but not church dogma. I could choose to be loyal to those I loved and not the "family mind." That is when I got results!

Most people believe that suffering is unavoidable. It is not. Suffering is optional. Suffering is self-imposed.

It is also important you understand that empathy does *not* mean joining in the suffering of another. We must *not* lower ourselves to the level of the person's frequency who is in the need of healing. It is our job to *lift* them out of the cause of their suffering into a state of joy. And for this, we must maintain our own connection to joy.

Addiction to Suffering

You could have all the right affirmations and all the right prayers, but if you have not handled the addiction to suffering, that could completely sabotage the healing. Perhaps you were raised in a church where they told you suffering was holy. Or even if you were not, it could come from past life memories of being Catholic, or Lutheran, etc.

Your parents and family members could have this addiction, and it could be influencing you. They could be suffering and might not like it if you are not suffering along with them! Some family members could actually think you do not love them if you are not suffering with them. Especially after a death in the family. Let's say they are sick and you happen to be happy. They might not be able to stand it. So, then you might unconsciously start suffering to make them comfortable.

Most people are not used to being happy all the time. That is unfamiliar. The mind tends to seek what is familiar. For sure, the belief in sin results in suffering. You may have been told in church were a sinner. But even if you were not told that, you probably were in recent past lives, which can still affect you.

The main thing to get is that guilt always demands punishment, and the main way we punish ourselves for our guilt is to suffer. In A Course in Miracles, Jesus has a lot to say about suffering. Basically, it says suffering is insane. Happiness and bliss have a healing effect on the body, so one has to know that God's will for us is perfect happiness.

Here are some passages from A Course in Miracles that clarify the causes and conditions of suffering:

Lesson # 136:

Sickness is a decision. It is not a thing that happens to you quite unsought, which makes you weak and brings you suffering. It is a choice you make, a plan you lay.

Lesson #41:

Depression is an inevitable consequence of separation. So are anxiety, worry, a sense of helplessness, misery and suffering.

Chapter 27 of the Text:

As long as you consent to suffer, you will be unhealed.

Lesson #53:

> If I see a world in which there is suffering, loss and death, it shows me I am seeing only a representation of my insane thoughts.

Chapter 16 of the Text:

> Only the wholly insane could look on death and suffering, sickness and despair and see it there.

Lesson #101:

> Pain is the cost of sin and suffering and can never be escaped if sin is real.

Lesson # 167:

> All sorrow, loss, anxiety, suffering and pain, even a sigh of weakness and slight discomfort, acknowledge death.

Chapter 24 of the Text:

> Suffering follows guilt.

Chapter 25 of the Text:

> And while you think that suffering and sin will bring you joy, so long will this be there for you. Nothing is harmful apart from what you wish.

Lesson #259:

> What else but sin could be the source of guilt, demanding punishment and suffering?

Chapter 27 of the Text:

While you believe that sin is real and punishment is just, salvation cannot be purchased but through suffering.

Manual for Teachers:

Who would choose suffering of any kind unless he thought it brought him something of value? And in your suffering of any kind, you see your own concealed desire to kill.

Lesson #164:

You can exchange all suffering for Joy this very day.

Chapter 13 of the Text:

Do not hide suffering from His sight but bring it gladly unto Him. Lay before His eternal sanity all your hurt. Suffering is not His creation.

Lesson #109

I rest in God. Here is the end of suffering for all the world.

Lesson #187:

Accept no suffering and you remove the thought of suffering.

Lesson # 249:

Forgiveness ends all suffering and loss. Forgiveness paints a picture of a world where suffering is over and loss becomes impossible and anger makes no sense.

Lesson # 284:

I can elect to change all thoughts that hurt. Then suffering of any kind is nothing but a dream.

Lesson # 285:

What would be the use of pain and what purpose would suffering fulfill if I accept my Holiness instead?

Chapter 10 of the Text:

Your Father created you wholly without pain and wholly without suffering of any kind. If you deny Him, you bring sin, pain and suffering into your own mind. It is blasphemous to perceive suffering.

Chapter 14 of the Text:

We are all joined in the Atonement. The miracle acknowledges the hope of happiness and release from suffering of any kind.

Chapter 16 of the Text:

True empathy does not mean to join in the suffering for that is the ego's interpretation...empathy is always used to form a special relationship in which suffering is shared. The Holy Spirit does not understand suffering.

Lesson # 337:

My sinlessness ensures me perfect peace, eternal safety, everlasting love, freedom forever from all thoughts of loss, complete deliverance from suffering and only happiness.

Lesson # 340:

I can be free of suffering today.

Markus on Choosing Joy Instead of Pain

Pain is something we all have experienced. Most of us would like to avoid pain as much as we can. But the fact is we will encounter pain and we will have a response to it. How do we respond to pain? Our negative response to pain, which is a mental and emotional reaction, I would call "suffering." Is it possible to end our experiences of pain without the response of suffering? What is this *power of decision* of our own mind? How do we access it? How do we harness it to heal ourselves and get out of the *effects* of pain?

There is a Lesson in A Course in Miracles that discusses this very response to pain that is what we need to master to liberate ourselves from suffering.

"I choose the Joy of God instead of pain."
(Lesson #190 in ACIM)

It is not the Will of our Creator for us to ever be in pain. Our will can be in conjunction with the Will of God to help us realize a Heaven state of being—in a totally pain-free existence of Immortal Life. There is a perfection in us that is totally pain-free. Our Spiritual Identity is untouched by pain. The acceptance of our Spiritual Identity requires that we align our mind with this higher reality free of pain, and not confuse our bodies with our Identity.

We have to forgive ourselves for this mistaken identification with physical stuff, and with a mind of "opposites"—life versus death—sickness versus health—pleasure versus pain. It is necessary to clean up this experience of pain, suffering, and conflict on earth. The world is actually composed of "neutral stuff." Can it all be aligned with the Will of God, which is Joy? Can we rise above the conflicts of our dualistic ego mind that projects pain, suffering and eventually death onto our life stream? To what focus will we give our Mind? Will we enter into our absolute and higher Mind, the realm of the Spirit Identification, that has transcended pain?

> *Here will you understand there is no pain. Here does the joy of God belong to you. This is the day when it is given you to realize the lesson that contains all of salvation's power. It is this: Pain is illusion; joy, reality. Pain is but sleep; joy is awakening. Pain is deception; joy alone is truth.*
>
> *And so again we make the only choice that ever can be made; we choose between illusions and the truth, or pain and joy, or hell and Heaven. Let our gratitude unto our Teacher fill our hearts, as we are free to choose our joy instead of pain, our holiness in place of sin, the peace of God instead of conflict, and the light of Heaven for the darkness of the world.*
> *(Lesson #190 in ACIM)*

This one choice we make is our major decision in Life. Will we liberate ourselves from the deception of pain and suffering, or will we perpetuate it with fear, anger and guilt?

Identification with Spirit, though, requires that we transcend the duality of thought, and the body. The ego's thought system itself is in a perpetual conflict; what is in conflict cannot be at peace; what is not in peace is at war with itself; and this results in pain and suffering. Given this situation, we need forgiveness in order to neutralize our experiences and memories of pain, suffering, conflict, and even death. We have to bring thought to silence. We have to bring the Mind to a stillness within that transcends thought as we have known it.

Even in this physical dimension it is possible to quiet the Mind through absolute and complete forgiveness. A Course in Miracles calls this the Atonement. We have forgiven everything and everyone, and we have accepted the forgiveness for ourselves as well. This is the doorway to the cessation of pain. We Identify with the non-physical nature of the Spirit, which is our Highest Reality. And this Identification transforms our Mind and our physical world into a balanced and Loving place—free of all grievances and judgments. This neutral place helps free us from pain. This is the Heaven State, or the Joy of God the Lesson invokes.

Joy and pain are mutually exclusive, and when we choose joy the pain must diminish. But the challenge is we have to make this choice in the midst of feeling some sort of pain. We have to "deny" the hold of pain over us, and choose another Reality instead. We must reach for thoughts and feelings of Joy in the middle of thoughts and feelings of pain. It is a Spiritual discipline to be able to do this, and to the ego it is "not normal." But it is a lot easier than thinking the negative thoughts that brought on the pain in the first place.

What we "think" and "feel" is up to us. We have dominion over our Mind. Therefore, it makes perfect sense that we can "choose the Joy of God instead of pain." A little willingness on our part is all that is needed to accept the fact that there is the "Joy of God" creating the Universe. It is a Life Force far greater than anything we have ever known. We can decide to tap into this Power. The Power of our decision is at our disposal. This Power can lift us out of all forms of pain and suffering, thus breaking our addiction to them.

6.

Anger and Sickness

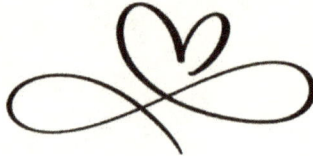

Anger is extremely damaging to your etheric substance and organs. It is also damaging to your relationships. When your relationships break down, your body breaks down. A Course in Miracles says, "Anger provokes separation, and communication ends separation," as well as, "Anger is never justified."

Anger and hatred are the most damaging emotions to your body because they close off the flow of life force energy to the body. Anger causes pain and sickness.

What is to be done about anger? I have written a lot about this in *Loving Relationships II*. Some of it is worth repeating here: Do not suppress anger; that is bad for your body. If you express it, that is bad for others. You need a way to handle anger. My teacher Babaji gave me the way. He said you should not suppress it, nor should you dump it on another. He said you must change the thought that causes anger and breathe out the energy. Are you willing to do that for the sake of your health? Can you remember to do this?

A lot of people might protest this technique, saying that the anger overtakes them quickly, before they can do anything about it. Train yourself how to handle anger. First, notice the feeling of anger coming up. Then immediately start breathing out the heavy energy and immediately try to change the negative thought coming up. DO NOT SPEAK WHEN YOU ARE ANGRY. Process your thoughts instead. Calm down first.

It is not hard if you put consciousness to it. What Markus and I do is this: We say "I am feeling ACTIVATED. The negative thought that is making me activated is_____." By doing this we are not stuffing anything. We are admitting we are charged up. But we don't have to be yelling or screaming. After we express the negative thought, we can breathe it out with a Breathwork session. If one cannot do that, one can take a cold shower or run around the block. Even drinking a glass of ice-cold water will help. Breathing out the charge is best. (It helps to have Liberation Breathing as a way of life so you know how to exhale anger and grow accustomed to observing your thoughts and changing them.) I like the word "activated" instead of using the word anger. The word anger has too much charge.

It is a bad habit to dump your anger on someone else, like your mate. A Course in Miracles says anger directed at someone is an attack and an attack is like a form of murder! (That is bad karma!) If you get angry at others and dump it on them, you are going to feel guilty. Remember that guilt truly can make you sick. Besides, it is probably not really *that person* who is making you angry. ACIM says you are never upset for the reason you think. In other words, it is usually an earlier similar event that is plugging you in.

I was conducting a marriage consultation once, and the husband told me he did not have to be the one to ask for forgiveness, because she, his wife, always started the argument. Therefore, (according to him) it was all her fault. I had to practically go over the whole Loving Relationships Training for him to understand that they both co-created that moment. He needed her to provoke him so he could have an excuse to fight and re-create his childhood and feel what was "familiar." She was, of course, just as responsible. We all co-create every moment. But he was stuck in blame and unwilling to see his part.

Imagine putting a little baby in a pressure cooker that was ON all the time. Would you do it? Of course not! So why would you do that to your body? You should always treat your body as kindly as you would a little baby's. I don't even let my body stay in the space of other people's anger. If anyone starts yelling and screaming, I leave. I am too sensitive. Of course, I look at my part in any dilemma, but I can look at my part of that outside the room and still protect my body. After all, we do have free will to put our bodies where we want.

I hope that now I am at peace enough so that all people around me feel that peace and want to be at peace in my presence. (That does not mean there is no excitement.) People who can maintain high levels of love and excitement and ecstasy without quickly blowing up afterward are getting somewhere. That probably means their subconscious is clear of anger. They can maintain peace in high energy. High energy tends to bring up anything unlike itself. You can tell a lot about people by watching them in high energy situations, especially afterward. They might go nuts for days afterward.

It is not true that you cannot control your anger. Who is in control of it? You are, of course, and thinking otherwise is a cop-out.

Here is what some gurus say on the subject:

Guru Mai:

"It is said that if you are a true ascetic, you are completely devoid of anger. If there is any trace of anger in you, you are called a scoundrel, not an ascetic. A great being will go to any extent to remove the fire of anger. The greatness of a Saddhu Monk is that he can drop something once he realizes he has it."

Dalai Lama:

"We lose control of our mind through hatred and anger. If our minds are dominated by anger, we will lose the best part of human intelligence – wisdom! Anger is one of the most serious problems facing the world today." (A Human Approach to World Peace" a pamphlet, page 12)

Mata Amritanandamayi (The Mother):

"Anger and impatience will always cause problems. Suppose you have a weakness of getting angry easily. Once you become normal again, go and sit in the family shrine room or in solitude and regret and repent your anger. Sincerely pray to your beloved deity or Mother Nature, seeking help to get rid of it. TRY TO MAKE YOUR OWN MIND AWARE OF THE BAD OUTCOME OF ANGER. When you are angry at someone, you lose all your mental balance. Your discriminative power completely stops functioning. You say whatever comes

into your mind and act accordingly. You may even utter crude words. By action and thinking with anger, you lose a lot of good energy. Become aware that these negative feelings will only pave the way for your own destruction! (Awaken Children, pp. 4-5) Amma also says anger makes you weak in every pore of your body.

What to Do During an Anger Attack

1. Do not yell at anyone else.

2. Lie down and breathe, pumping out your anger on the exhale. (It helps to know how to do Liberation Breathing.)

3. If that does not work, walk or run around the block until calm. Take a cold shower and drink ice water.

4. When you calm down, remind yourself of these two lines from A Course in Miracles:

   A. "You will attack what does not satisfy you to avoid seeing that you created it."
   B. "Beware of the temptation to perceive yourself as unfairly treated."

5. This means you created the result at which you are angry. You somehow wanted it, needed it, or are addicted to it, so try to get enlightened about this fact and see your part! (What is your payoff? What *benefit* are you getting out of this that is neurotic?)

6. Express yourself sanely now.
   A. "I felt angry because _____." Or even better: "I got activated because _____."
   B. "I see now that I had the thought _____, and that thought attracted this situation."
   C. "I apologize for this, and I want to repent and make amends."

7. Do the process recommended above by Mata Amritanandamayi in a holy area. A holy area might be a room or special part of a room where one has an altar to spiritual masters, or any other place indoors or out, in which you feel at peace.

8. If you are not completely calm, write down your feelings of anger and then burn the paper.

9. If you feel none of the above works, call a friend who is more enlightened than you are at the time to get help processing. Ask for a Liberation Breathing session as soon as possible.

10. Do a Truth Process such as, "The reason I do not want to forgive is _____." (Usually seeing your part in the situation dilutes the problem if you are telling the truth.)

11. Remember that forgiveness is the key to happiness and health.

12. Remember that behind every grievance, there is a miracle.

13. Remember that anger is one of the causes of aging and death. (It is *not* worth it.)

Follow Catherine Ponder's steps to forgiveness:

A. You forgive them.
B. You forgive yourself.
C. Allow them to forgive you.
D. Give up all desire to punish and get even.
E. Restore good harmony as before the upset.

Sometimes we get angry that we have a symptom in our body—especially if it does not go away. The problem is this: anger keeps the symptom stuck and in place. Anger will ruin your health. It makes you vibrate at a low level, and it can destroy the former spiritual work you have done on yourself.

If you want to be healthy and stay healthy, give up your anger. That includes all anger: suppressed anger, covert anger, overt anger, even irritation. People think they can get by with irritation and that that is okay. ACIM says that below every irritation is a veil of hate! You cannot let in God's love (which would heal you) if you are angry.

Anger is due to lack of forgiveness. When you forgive everyone and everything 100%, that is when your anger will dissolve. It is not that you can't forgive someone; it is that you won't. Not forgiving is due to a stubborn refusal. Forgiveness is the key to happiness and the key to health. It has been said that when there is an illness, there is a forgiveness problem. Most people go to the grave with an accumulation of non-forgiveness.

WHAT YOU HAVE NOT FORGIVEN, YOU ATTRACT. Let's say you have not forgiven your father for leaving you as a child. Then you will go on creating mates that leave you and you might keep doing that over and over until you forgive.

In Liberation Breathing we always do a forgiveness check. We ask what level of forgiveness a client has on their mother, their father, their ex and themselves. Ten is total forgiveness, zero is none. Five is obviously half. People get very low scores. They might get five or less on a parent. If they get eight, that is better, but not good enough. ACIM says if you have not forgiven at 10 (100%) you have not really forgiven at all. (Did you get that?)

Lack of forgiveness = anger. Anger will destroy your body. It will definitely destroy your relationships. Who wants to be around an angry person? You don't like to be in the presence of angry people, so why would you think its ok for you to be angry, without driving people away?

7.

Guilt and Sickness

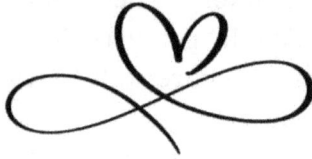

Guilt demands punishment. In your ego's mind, you believe that is so. One of the ways we punish ourselves when we feel guilty is to get sick. We attack our bodies with an illness, pain, or injury that we make up.

A Course in Miracles says that guilt is not only not of God, but an attack on God! It says it is a sure sign that your thinking is *unnatural*. This is all explained in a section called *The Ego's Use of Guilt*. The Course also says that if you have guilt, you are walking the carpet of death! That means that we think we must eventually die as a form of punishment for our guilt, especially since we think we are such sinners! We therefore kill ourselves with our own thoughts by squeezing out our life force.

Sometimes, you may not even realize you are guilty until you get a symptom. In this way, the symptoms serve you to make you aware of the guilt. By the way, with INNOCENCE you can ward off any disease.

A few years back, I developed a lot of tension because of having to fire someone. It is the dreaded part of my job as a leader. I realized the tension was due to the guilt, but I could not seem to shake it, so I discussed it with someone more spiritually advanced at the time. That teacher said, "Your problem as a leader is that you don't ever let people fall on their faces." He made it clear to me that some people set it up that way to finally learn their lessons. In effect, they "fire" themselves! I appreciated that teaching, and so I did it. He helped me to see I was innocent for what I had to do.

Reading A Course in Miracles helps you become re-grounded in your innocence. It says you can have forgiveness in the Holy Instant because God does not make your sins real. The Holy Instant is one's choice to accept the energy of love over fear and unity over separation. *Sins* means your "case" or your "issues" or your "mistakes." God knows that your "case" is just ego, which is not real. This may seem like an advanced concept if you have not read much of A Course in Miracles. Another way to say this is, "Your ego is a nightmare that you are temporarily experiencing." You think you are separate (ego), but that is not real. You can't be separate from God. When your child has a nightmare, for example, you don't make *it* real, nor does God make our nightmares real. It is important to keep studying A Course in Miracles until you finally understand this point.

Along with the idea of guilt, one must beware of the danger of carrying "deep, dark secrets." This is like having inside you a festering sore full of guilt, which you pretend you do not have, and you pretend it does not affect your body. This keeps eating away at you—no doubt about it. You must be willing to tell someone if you have some deep secret about which you feel guilty. That was one of the whole ideas of going to a priest. However, confession in the church has in many cases been used to make one feel even more guilty. It might be better to share your dark secret with someone you really trust. Get it off your chest.

An acquaintance of mine was killed in a small plane crash. I had trouble understanding why he had crashed because he was quite enlightened. I wanted to know what went wrong with his mind to attract that fate. I begged one of my teachers (a seer) to tell me. He was reluctant, but after he saw the insomnia I suffered because of that death, he finally told me that this man had a deep, dark secret. I was later surprised to learn he was a very secretive person. In the end, the guilt he held and concealed did him in. I started teaching my students to confess their deep secrets. One girl finally told the group her father was in the Mafia! Her whole life changed after that. She became younger and very powerful in her own right.

Once I did something I thought was stupid, and I could not let go of it. One friend knew about it, but it was not enough for me to tell just him. He realized I needed a ceremony, so he put me in his car and drove me out into the woods to meet a recluse friend of his. He told me to go into the shack and confess this thing to his friend, the recluse. I did it. I have no idea who that person was or is to this day, but he was very loving. He did not know or care who I was either. He heard what I said and loved me and did not bat an eye. He thought it was trivial. I obviously got over the whole ordeal by confessing and cannot even remember what it was about now.

Years later I found myself with a silly habit that I was embarrassed about. I was a public figure by then and I did not want to tell anyone. Then I remembered the friend who had driven me to see the recluse, so I went to see him again. He was hanging out in his kitchen with another friend from San Diego. Now, that guy was the opposite of a recluse. He was gregarious and wealthy and all that, and he was "cool." I decided this was the right moment and I blurted out my embarrassing bad habit. They both looked at me and said in unison, "So what!" before moving on to something a lot more interesting. The next day the habit disappeared from my life forever.

Find someone to talk to, even a stranger if there isn't anyone else. Try it! We all have some past life guilt, birth trauma guilt for hurting our mothers, religious guilt, and guilt for things we did in this life. The separation was our original guilt. We thought we were separate from the life force (God); however, as I said, it is impossible to be separate from our Source of Life.

While guilt may be attractive, the mind and body will suffer. A Course in Miracles says that THE BELIEF IN SIN IS A REQUEST FOR DEATH! (The ego tells us we deserve death.) Love and guilt cannot co-exist. Peace and guilt cannot co-exist. Remember that guilt is not only not of God, it is an attack on God. To the ego, there is no escape from guilt. It tells us that if we dare to think we are innocent then we are really guilty! Those who hold grievances will suffer guilt. If we yield to guilt, we are deciding against health and happiness. To heal ourselves, we must know and accept that we are innocent. Otherwise, we will keep the condition as a punishment for our guilt. Innocence can ward off any disease. The blanket of guilt we lay on our bodies will kill us. We become addicted to feeling bad. Guilt can manifest as psychosomatic diseases, accident proneness, and suicidal behavior. One must decide to either cling to guilt and get the "juice" from it or give it up. No healing can occur until the right decision is made. The way to escape pain, is guiltlessness. Our holiness is our salvation; it is the end of guilt. The guiltless mind does not and cannot suffer. Recovery from guilt may include confession, forgiveness, penance, renewal of spiritual principles, good works, selfless service, and humanitarian efforts.

The Addiction to Guilt

All your problems of pain and sickness originate with guilt. Somewhere in A Course in Miracles it says that guilt is not only not of God, it is an attack on God! Our original guilt stems from the fact that we think we separated from God by taking on a body. Guilt always demands punishment so we then proceed to punish ourselves unconsciously by creating problems, pain, sickness, and ultimately death.

Then we assume it is somehow wrong to give up guilt. A Course in Miracles says you have to pass through the temptation of thinking that if you go for innocence, then you are REALLY guilty. This is the trap most people never ever get out of. If you think you are a sinner, your guilt will be everlasting!

People create their own hell while alive because of all their guilt. ACIM says "Hell is what the ego makes of the present."

There can be past life guilt/guilt for hurting your mother at birth/guilt about making mistakes and religious guilt. This chapter is mostly applies to your original guilt because that is the deepest.

You might not think you are guilty and maybe you never think about it. However, the guilt is buried in your subconscious and if you have any pain or sickness, that is a result of the guilt that you may not be feeling. You are not feeling it—but you are acting it out! Without guilt the ego has no life. It is our job to give up (transcend) the ego. The fact is that we need to know that we are completely innocent in order to be completely healed!

Lesson #13

❖ "It is guilt that has driven you insane."
❖ "The acceptance of guilt was the beginning of the separation."
❖ "If you are to retain guilt, as the ego insists, you cannot be You."

Lesson #14

❖ "Guilt is always disruptive. Anything that engenders fear is divisive. The ego is the symbol of guilt."
❖ "Guilt is interference, not salvation and serves no useful function at all."

Lesson #15

❖ "Guilt must lead to the belief in hell and always does."
❖ "Guilt remains the only thing that hides the Father for guilt is an attack upon His Son."

Lesson #16

❖ "The appeal of hell lies in the terrible attraction of guilt."

Lesson #18

❖ "You have displaced your guilt to your body from your mind."

Lesson #19

- ❖ "While guilt remains attractive, the mind will suffer."
- ❖ "The attraction of guilt produces fear of love."
- ❖ "When the attraction of guilt holds sway, peace is not wanted."
- ❖ "From the ego comes sin, guilt and death. No one can die unless he chooses death. What seems to be fear of death, is really its attraction."

Lesson #26

- ❖ "Guilt asks for punishment and the request is granted."

Lesson #27

- ❖ "Wish not to make yourself a symbol of guilt for you will not escape death. Sickness is the witness to guilt and death.
- ❖ "Sickness is but a little death."

Lesson #30

- ❖ "Guilt is the sole cause of pain in any form."
- ❖ "As long as you feel guilty, you are listening to the voice of the ego."

Chapter 13

- ❖ "Peace and guilt are antithetical."
- ❖ "Love and guilt cannot co-exist and to accept one is to deny the other."

Lesson #15

- ❖ "The attraction of guilt opposes the attraction of God."

Lesson #16

❖ "The appeal of hell lies only in the terrible attraction of guilt."

Lesson # 24

❖ "Specialness is the lack of trust in anyone but yourself. Death is enthroned as savior. Crucifixion is now redemption. Such is guilt's attraction."

Lesson #25

❖ "To the extent to which you value guilt, to that extent will you perceive a world in which attack is justified."

Lesson #70

❖ "All guilt is solely an invention of your own mind."

Lesson #12

❖ "The undoing of guilt is an essential part of the Holy Spirit's teaching."

Lesson #13

❖ "Forgiveness takes all guilt away."

❖ "The Holy Spirit seeks to remove all guilt from your mind that you may remember Your Father."

❖ "Only in your guiltlessness can you be happy."

Lesson #14

❖ "There is no guilt in you because God is blessed in His Son and the Son is blessed in Him. The burden of guilt is heavy; but God would not have you bound by it."

❖ "Your only calling here is to devote yourself with active willingness to the denial of guilt."

Lesson #16
❖ "The Holy Instant is the most helpful aid in protecting you from the attraction of guilt."

Lesson #18
❖ "You have been told to bring guilt to holiness."
❖ "Never attempt to overlook your guilt before you ask the Holy Spirit's help. That is His function. Your part is to offer Him a little willingness."

Lesson #19
❖ "You want salvation, not the pain of guilt. The end of guilt is in your hands."

Lesson #22
❖ "The escape from guilt was given to the Holy Spirt as His Purpose."

Lesson # 39
❖ "Your holiness means the end of all guilt and therefore the end of hell."

Lesson #58
❖ "From my holiness does the perception of the real world come. Having forgiven, I no longer see myself as guilty. I can accept the innocence that is the truth about me. There is nothing that is apart from this joy. My holiness saves me from all guilt."

Lesson #62

❖ "Forgiveness will remove all sense of weakness, strain, fatigue from your mind. It will take away all fear, pain and guilt."

Lesson #140

❖ "Atonement does not heal the sick, but takes away the guilt that makes sickness possible."

Lesson #157

❖ "Through your transfiguration is the world redeemed and joyfully released from guilt."

Lesson #162 ("I am as God created me.")

❖ "Yours is the right to perfect holiness you now accept. With this acceptance is salvation brought to everyone. Who could despair when perfect joy is yours available and the remedy for grief, misery, and complete escape from guilt."

Lesson #192

❖ "Forgiveness is the means by which the fear of death is overcome because it holds no fierce attraction now and guilt is gone!

Manual for Teachers

❖ "Spirit's guidance is to let yourself be absolved of guilt. That is the essence of the Atonement."

8.

Fear and Sickness

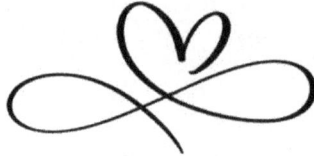

A Course in Miracles says all healing is essentially the release from fear. It also says only two emotions exist: love and fear. Love is God. That won't make us sick. Fear is ego. That *will* make us sick.

Fear may seem beyond our control, but it is not. Fear is self-controlled. We *are* responsible for what we think. When we have fear, ACIM says it is a sure sign we have allowed our minds to miscreate. When we are fearful, we have chosen wrongly. When we ask God to take away our fear, we imply that it is not our responsibility. We must ask instead for help with the conditions that have brought our fears about. A condition that produces fear, according to ACIM, is our desire to remain separate from God. Our fear prevents us from letting the Holy Spirit be in charge. If we let the Holy Spirit be in charge, no fear will exist. Fear is, then, a result of our "control number."

A Course says that attempting to master fear is useless because that gives fear more power. The only way to overcome fear is to master love. Fear comes from thoughts. By choosing loving thoughts, we are rejecting fear. In ACIM, Jesus offers these steps to release fear:

1. Know first that this is fear.
2. Fear arises from lack of love.
3. The only remedy for lack of love is perfect Love.
4. Perfect love is the Atonement.

In ACIM, the Atonement means allowing the Holy Spirit to correct your wrong thinking.

Here is a powerful quotation from ACIM: *"I (Jesus) know it (fear) does not exist; but you do not. You believe in the power of what does not exist."*
What He is saying is that fear does not really exist, because fear is the ego, and the ego is separation, and separation does not exist. We are not separate from the Source, but we have made separation seem real, we have made the ego seem real, and we have made fear seem real. As long as we think we are separate from God, we WILL have fear.
Anytime we are sick, we are replacing God with the ego. The part of our body that suffers is where we are storing our ego (fear) and pushing out God. That is why ACIM says that "sickness is idolatry." It goes so far as to say that when you are sick, you are trying to kill God!
The body cannot act wrongly unless it is responding to mis-thoughts. Our thoughts alone are what cause us pain and sickness. It is a fundamental error to believe the body is creating illness. ACIM tells us over and over that if we are sick, we are withdrawing from God and are spiritually deprived. It repeatedly states that all forms of illness are physical expressions of fear.

There is the fear that causes sickness, and then there is the fear of healing. The reason healing is a threat is that it means *we are responsible* for our thoughts. The mind makes the decision to be sick. All illness is mental illness. Most people do not want to face this fact. They would rather blame something outside themselves; it seems easier. But if we keep blaming things outside ourselves and shirking responsibility for our thoughts, how can we ever heal ourselves?

Some people are afraid of healing because they have chosen sickness as a way of life to get attention and they fear losing that attention and getting depressed. They must be willing to give up the position of victim and reclaim their power.

People are often very afraid of the miracle healings they say they want. They may pray for a miracle but are terrified of that. This is because experiencing a miracle would change their whole reality. ACIM recommends that we clearly understand how to pray for healing. It recommends that we do not pray for a miracle healing of cancer or arthritis to happen overnight. We have too much fear of that kind of a miracle, too much fear of that much light, of that much reality shifting that fast. We most likely would not let it happen unless we were in the presence of Jesus or Mary at the shrine. People may be more willing to allow a miracle at holy places (such as a shrine like Lourdes) because they feel safer and can better sense the presence of Mary or Jesus. But we can know that we stand on holy ground and that they are right there with us at any time.

In ACIM, Jesus says to pray for the *removal of the fear of healing* first. After all, the Holy Spirit is not going to *add* to our fear! If we are terrified of miracles,

He is not going to scare the hell out of us with one. We must prepare our mind. We must be ready for miracles. We must be over the fear of healing before we will let it happen.

Misery, pain, suffering, and death; we are all used to them. We are also addicted to them. What we are truly afraid of is life, God, and love. This fear makes us hang onto conditions that bring us down in energy to a state that is more familiar than all the energy we would have in a state of absolute, pristine, and perfect health or in the incredible light-energy of a miracle.

We are so confused that we actually think God kills people. If God is energy, then in that way of thinking, energy kills people. So, we are also terrified of energy. And yet the truth is, the energy of God can heal us completely. But we must get our mind straight first or we will stop the whole process. ACIM says no one is sick or dies without his own consent.

Jesus said that the Atonement cures all sickness. The Atonement is total and complete forgiveness of everything. It takes away all fear and guilt. When there is no more fear, there is no more pain. To be symptomless we must give up all fear. What is our fear of giving up fear? The answer is that we would probably be in ecstasy. Ecstasy does not have to be scary; it is just unfamiliar. People fear that something bad will happen, but they even are afraid that something good will happen!

How do we give up fear?

    a. We must be willing to find the negative thought causing the fear.

    b. We must be willing to give up that thought.

c. We must then turn it all over to the Holy Spirit.

Usually there is some "payoff" to keeping the negative thought or the condition. There is a neurotic benefit that we are getting. We might maintain a sickness, or a condition, because it gets us attention that we would not get otherwise. Or it gives us an excuse to stay home. We may get out of something we do not want to do as a result of being sick. We may have a partner or family member at our disposal as a result of our fear.

Once you notice the fear, you say, "The fear I have of being free of this condition is _____." What comes up for you? Then you have to turn this around. You have to be willing to think differently and let go of this fear. For example, "My fear of really being in my power is that people will be jealous of me." You have to think differently. "My power is helpful to others; others are inspired when I am in my power."

You also have to clear your payoff. "The benefit I get from keeping this condition is _____." It could be, "I get to stay small and not be in my power. I get to be lazy and not work too hard staying small. I have more time to myself." Giving this up might look like this: "I love being in my power, and so do others like it. I enjoy all the opportunities that come to me being in my power."

"Turning the matter over to the Holy Spirit" can mean different things to different people. Basically, it means we are trusting in a Higher Source that is benevolent to our greatest good. The Great Unknown is on our side. We may not "know how" to make a shift, heal a condition, or be free of an addiction. But there is trust we have in things turning around in our favor. There is a God or a Life Force that wants the best for us, and we have the faith that this Force will move things in our direction for the better. This is necessary in overcoming fear. We trust in a Higher Power to set right all the things in our life that have "gone off." This energy puts us on the right course, and re-establishes our flow of infinite well-being. In this flow, when we are really with it and we know it, there is nothing to fear.

9.

The Unconscious Death Urge

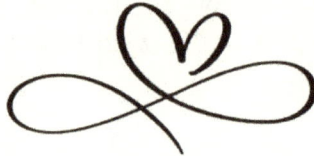

One of the *main* causes of sickness and symptoms is what we call *the unconscious death urge*. This is the ego in its worse form. It includes thoughts like the following:

- ❖ The thought "I am separate from God"
- ❖ The belief that "death is inevitable"
- ❖ Our programming from society and family about death
- ❖ Our family patterns on disease, aging, and death
- ❖ The invalidation of our personal divinity
- ❖ Addictions and bad habits leading to aging and death
- ❖ Any anti-life thoughts
- ❖ Our secret wish to die because we hate our life
- ❖ False religious theology
- ❖ Past-life memories of dying

All of this is like a *conglomerate* in our subconscious mind. It will ruin us until we take charge of our mind and clear it. This can be done.

If we constantly affirm "death is inevitable," death is the result we will get. The way to create death is to create sickness and aging so we can die. In Proverbs 18:21 KJV Jesus said, "Death and life are in the power of the tongue." That means that what we *say* is what we *get* in our body. We are at cause over our body. Our body is like a computer printout; we are the programmer.

Most people believe that death is beyond their control. Some blame it on God. But if we believe that God controls our death, we are making God a murderer! Others blame something out there in the universe, as if "something" is out to get them. If that is the case, it is impossible to walk around and relax. Our physical body will break down with the tension of wondering when "it" (death) is going to get us. When we try to live while having the thought that death is inevitable, it is like trying to drive a car forward while shifted in reverse with the brakes on. The car will break down. Our body will break down.

Our physical body is our most valuable possession, but have you noticed that people take better care of their cars and houses than they do their bodies? People allow their bodies to be destroyed, sometimes easily, without protest.

It is our *mind* that kills our body. Therefore, all death is suicide! A Course in Miracles says, "Death is a result of a thought called the Ego." People use their egos to kill themselves. If we believe that death is inevitable, we are in the process of dying right now. We are programming it right now. If we heal one disease and do not change that thought, we will just make up another one to kill ourselves. That is why Leonard Orr said, "All healing is temporary until you heal death." ACIM says, "No one can die unless he chooses death." (ACIM; Text; Chapter 19; Section IV C; ¶1)

What is the point of learning to heal yourself if you keep trying to kill yourself with your subconscious limiting thoughts?

The instant we forgot who we were and created the fall (separation-ego), death became our punishment for that "sin." The belief in sin is the request—the self-command—for punishment and death. Once we accept the idea that we are separate from God, our Source Energy, it is all downhill. We will have thoughts about not having any power, being weak, not be able to heal ourselves, and perhaps not deserving life.

The "deathist mentality" is predominant in our society. We are taught that *death is inevitable*. This belief system is like many others; participating in it makes us feel safe, in this case even while it is killing us. This is a false sense of safety. When you get outside belief systems, you start experiencing mastery and go to *direct knowing*. And that is thrilling. Are you willing to change your belief system?

Most people cannot imagine wanting to live forever and giving up their death urge, because they are in so much pain. What they do not realize is that the reason they are in pain in the first place is because of their death urge. (It's a Catch-22.) One must figure this out.

Your death urge could be operating in many areas of your life. The obvious one is your body. However, you might also be "killing off" your relationships, your business, your friendships, and what-not. You may be losing money in investments because you are killing them off. Never underestimate the power of the ego and the unconscious death urge.

It is important to see that the death urge causes disease, not the other way around. People think they get sick, age, and then die. What they really do is die in their minds, which causes sickness and aging.

One main point of A Course in Miracles is that hell is what the ego makes of the present. We create our own hell with our ego, and then, after misusing our power and creating hell, we think we deserve to die. (Or we may even want to die!) In our minds, death becomes the only way out. And according to our egos, we don't think we deserve to live even if we wanted to! Usually, we don't want to live because we turned our life into hell: pain, misery, suffering, and aging. A Course spends a long time showing us our "descent into hell." To get out of all this we must become a master—and that is the whole point of our life in the first place!

The main reason it is so important to understand the above is that we create illnesses because of our unconscious death urge. ACIM says: "All illness is ALWAYS the wish to die and overcome the Christ." If you want to be healed, you must handle and heal your unconscious death urge. Unfortunately, many people are into the "waiting to die syndrome" thinking they will be in bliss in Heaven. You need to know that consciousness seeks its own level after you die. Then you will have to come back and go through it all again until you get enlightened. Why not ask for enlightenment in this life? Why not ask to be as God created us:

You are as God created you. All else but this one thing is folly to believe. In this one thought is everyone set free. In this one truth are all illusions gone. In this one fact is sinlessness proclaimed to be forever part of everything, the central core of its existence and its guarantee of immortality. (ACIM; Workbook; Lesson #191; ¶4)

You may ask, "Why would anyone ever want to live forever?" You would only ask that if you did not love your life. Of course. we are not talking about living a long time in an old, decrepit body. We are talking about the ability to live as long as you choose WHILE improving your body, for a mission of Divine Service. There are immortal masters. I have met some.

All healing is temporary until you heal death. We could teach you, for example how to heal cancer (cancer is a battle between the life urge and the death urge and the cells are confused), but if you do not heal your death urge, you will just make up a new way to kill yourself. We have written a whole book on this subject: *Physical Immortality: How to Overcome Death.* You can get it here: bit.ly/ImmortalRay

10.

Past Lives and Sickness

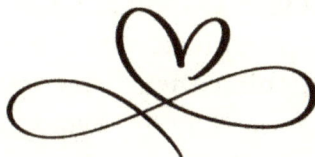

I was not aware of the effects of past lives when I was young; I did not even know about the subject! It was certainly not something discussed in church (even though there are references in the Bible about those who lived "before" as someone else). Nor was this topic discussed in medicine when I studied nursing.

When I moved to California in the 1970s I was compelled to read books by authors such as Edgar Cayce who opened me up to past life ideas. And after a while, I started looking at the subject more closely. In a session one day a client of mine remembered being in a war in Ireland in a past life. She began speaking with a perfect Irish accent. Later I asked her if she had ever been to Ireland, and she said no. I asked her if she had ever studied Irish dialect and she said no. I asked her if she remembered speaking to me in long paragraphs in Irish with a perfect Irish accent without hesitation. She was able to remember scenes, but not the Irish speaking part.

After that, I began to have more past life memories in my own sessions. I clearly saw scenes from other eras that I had never glimpsed in a movie or read about. The styles of furniture and architecture were different from anything I had known in my current life. What always amazed me was that I had such strong emotions while having those memories. They were so spontaneous and real that I knew I could not be making them up. I started paying attention.

After my first visit to India, I began to have past life memories frequently. It was as if my guru Babaji was deliberately pushing them into my mind to be cleared. There was no way to avoid this clearing, whether I liked it or not. This has gone on for years now. As I got stronger, more difficult ones came up. One year my guru Shastriji put a tourniquet on my left arm and shouted mantras to my third eye for several minutes. So many past lives came up that year I could hardly believe it! The next year he did the same thing on the other arm and worse ones came up that year. The following year he put a tourniquet on both arms and shouted mantras again. Need I tell you how hard that year was. I am forever grateful for this however. It cleared me of a lot of stuff.

Now I can relate to many stories told by clients with illnesses they couldn't seem to heal until they came to us for a Liberation Breathing session. Unquestionably, I can say that Breathwork with a past life regression did the trick. I am happy that this kind of healing is now being adequately and professionally researched. I recommend that everyone read the book *Other Lives, Other Selves* by Dr. Roger Woolger. His book is a must for all Breathworkers and healers. It is hard to put down. The studies he has done are awesome and must have made a huge impact on the field of psychology by now. In the first chapter, Dr. Woolger acknowledges that he was a skeptic who encountered past lives ONLY after he himself started Breathwork.

On page 100, Dr. Woolger states:

The body and its various aches, pains, and dysfunction is a living psychic history when read correctly. Even though the physical ailment may have very specific origins in a person's current life, I have found more and more that there are certain layers to every major syndrome of physical illness, accident, or weakness. The existence of a past life level of physical problems has been confirmed over and over again in the cases I have seen.

On page 101:

A woman in her early forties relived an unfulfilled life as a woman in the pioneer days which ended tragically when a horse and trap overturned, she broke her back and died when she was twenty-seven in that life. In this life, at age twenty-seven, she was in the hospital with a very serious kidney infection which they could not properly diagnose, and she nearly died. ... The pain was terrible and was in the same place where she had broken her back in the other life.

On page 143, he describes his work with phobias:

Although many phobias do, indeed, arise in this life, it seems to be the case that almost everyone has some deep fear that will not be explained. Whether it be fear of spiders, wild animals, fire, water, heights, crowds, knives, dark places, and so on. I have consistently found that behind that fear lies a specific and detailed story of a past-life trauma. In sessions, people remember deaths from poisonous insects, from spiders, snakes, sharks, and more. Many who fear heights recall deaths from being thrown off cliffs, falling from planes in recent wars, etc.

On page 171:

Increasingly, in practicing psychotherapy from a past life perspective, I am convinced that the likelihood of a cure depends on whether or not I am able to guide my client to the crucial or key story from his or her past lives.

His book also contains stories about how gynecological problems related to past lives of sexual abuse and rape. There are many detailed accounts about how these ancient traumas relate to present-day frigidity and lack of orgasm in women.

Clearing Past Lives in a Breathwork Session

In a Liberation Breathing session we take an extensive life review of a person, all the way back to their birth, in order to look at where they might be holding memories of traumas and subconscious negative beliefs formed about themselves, family members, partners, and all areas of their life experiences.

Sometimes a person has had a fairly easy life, with loving parents and a good childhood, and everything in their current life is supportive of happy outcomes. However, there is an issue nagging them that cannot be explained in their history. This is usually an indication that there is a past life that was incomplete, and the source of a problem, such as a pervading sense of guilt, or fear, or anger, that is lingering in their mind, which they cannot seem to shake. A person may hold in their mind a "personal lie," their most negative thought about themselves, like "I am bad." But nothing in this life indicates they did anything bad, or had the overbearing disapproval from a parent that would result in such a thought. In this case, usually, there is a past life incident that is being dragged over that could be giving them a sense of something "bad" in themselves.

In these cases, we actually ask the person if they have had any past life regressions. If not, we ask them to recall a time in which they felt "bad" that may come from an ancient memory from a life gone by. Usually, with the right atmosphere of openness and non-judgment, the past life will emerge during the Breathwork, and the person can see with incredible detail an incident in which they formed that feeling. They see where and when the self-judgment was formed, that carried-over emotion that had no explanation from events in their current life. We ask them to breathe into this memory, and look at as much detail as possible. Sometime there was a death, either of themselves or someone else with whom they were closely involved. They look at the whole scene as if they are there, hovering above it, observing it unfolding before them.

In the case of a violent death, we ask them to sink into the action of the scene, and observe the death—sometimes their own. They can "send light" to the situation, forgive themselves and all parties involved, and let peace rest upon all things as they breathe into re-experiencing the scene. But this time they know they will live, and go on. In this way the judgments of the incident, such as this thought formed—"I am bad"—are forgiven and released.

You would be surprised how much this revisitation in a Breathwork session helps to clear a person's psyche of heavy thoughts. They need not carry the guilt or the sadness any more from a life that is not even here now. Any time we can let go of baggage we are carrying from any part of our past is very liberating to our present. This may be from a past life, a memory long ago, that was so traumatic we were not able to forget it. Liberation Breathing is a great way to help release and neutralize these kinds of memories. It is very effective in clearing people of the negative feelings they bring over from past lives.

11.

Your Relationship with Your Symptoms

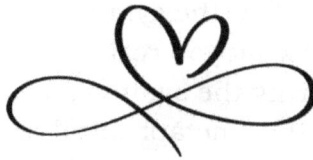

When you develop symptoms or a disease, you might react to the situation in several different ways:

- ❖ *You might deny it is going on at all.*
- ❖ *You might acknowledge it but avoid it.*
- ❖ *You might be angry at the situation.*
- ❖ *You might fight it and get in a battle with your mind.*
- ❖ *You might resist it.*
- ❖ *You might hate yourself for it.*
- ❖ *You might continually complain about it.*
- ❖ *You might continually worry about it.*
- ❖ *You might get obsessed with it.*
- ❖ *You might get depressed about it.*

❖ *You might overdose with food, liquor, or drugs to suppress it.*

❖ *You might get terrified of it.*

❖ *You might mistakenly think it has more power than you do.*

It is extremely tempting to take one of these approaches, especially if the symptoms stick around. The trouble is that "what you resist persists," so these approaches only fortify the symptoms.

Remember the metaphysical principle that what you think about expands so, the more you dwell on it in a negative way, the worse it will get. True, it *is* hard not to dwell on it negatively, especially when it is painful. But it will get more painful when you dwell on it! Denying it is not good either. You need to learn from it and take the necessary action to change.

Then you must get a hold of your mind. A Course in Miracles says that "The physician is the mind of the patient himself." This means you are your own doctor; you created the symptom, and you can uncreate it. But you must start by giving up the above tempting tendencies, and you must develop a loving relationship with your symptom or disease. How do you do that? Ah, yes, that is the trick!

First, acknowledge it as a blessing in that it is there to show you that your mind is *off*. It is there to teach you something important. It is there to teach you that your mind needs correction. It is there to get your attention. When you are experiencing a symptom in the body, you tend to start a battle with it. There is another way.

Second, ask the symptom what it is trying to tell you. Or have a friend ask you this question: "If your symptom could talk, what would it say to you?" It is not acceptable to say, "I don't know." You *do* know. The answer is within. Your partner or friend should not accept that answer. They must then say to you, "If you did know, what would it be?" "I don't know" comes from not looking. For exact information on the cause of this condition, do the Ultimate Truth Process found in Chapter 20. This is a very, very important step in self-analysis; if you want permanent healing, you must know the *cause.*

Third, try the techniques in this book. If the symptom or disease does not shift after self-analysis (the Truth Process and Breathwork, for example), you need much more understanding of the framework in this book and the techniques given later. Go to a Liberation Breathing practitioner for example, and find out why you do not want to be healed.

Fourth, remember that the sickness is the "cure in process". This means you take the attitude of experiencing your condition as a purging of a negative thought or construct, rather than as something stuck. Taking this attitude is very important; it's the basis for your healing. You must train yourself to remember that your body is trying to "spit out" the effects of the negative thought that caused it. Your body is attempting to cure itself when you have symptoms. You need to mentally cooperate with this healing process. If you fight it, ignore it, or react in one or more of the negative ways mentioned at the beginning of this chapter, you will only add negative mental mass.

12.

Attitude and Frame of Mind

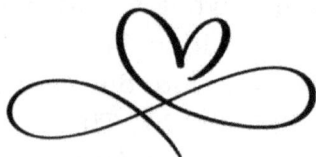

In my opinion, the hardest part of being sick (besides feeling terrible, of course) is the worry that the condition will never end. So often one is tempted to think, "What if I don't get over this?" This fear can escalate to the point that you start thinking you will not get over it. At that point, you may even start feeling like your body controls you instead of you controlling it.

When you have overwhelming fear, you forget that you control your body with your mind, and you start thinking that your body or disease controls you—that it is more powerful than you. Then the situation worsens because you feel helpless. You are losing it now, and you must take drastic action to realize that *you* are in charge. Your body is never the cause. You are. Your mind is. If you don't correct your mind at this point, you might become paralyzed with fear to the point that the body's automatic healing system literally shuts down. Or you could end up crystallizing the symptoms into something very solid. Therefore, it is important to get through this danger by having the thought, *This too will pass.*

A person may go from doctor to doctor or from healer to healer while none of them can help because part of the person's mind is trying to prove the condition cannot be healed. That way the person can continue to hate God for his or her plight and remain angry rather than changing. Of course, people who "need" their anger for this reason, rarely admit it. It is their little secret. Or they could be in total denial about their war against God. If one were healed and remained healed, felt fantastic, and everything was working, what would there be to get angry at? Some people do not want to give up their need to blame.

If you create the sickness or symptoms because you want attention, you may not want to be healed either, because you would lose all the attention. This is another trap! If you create the symptom as a way of suffering because you believe that you *must* suffer, you might also set yourself up not to be healed. If you create the sickness or symptoms as a way of punishing yourself for something, you will probably set yourself up not to be healed because you still think you need more punishment.

When you finally see no more value in the pain, suffering, and self-punishment, you will spontaneously heal yourself or finally manifest the right doctor or healer to help you do the trick. ACIM says: "The outcome is what the patient decides." It will spontaneously become obvious to you what you need to do or where you need to go or with whom you need to be to end your ailment. God is ready when you are. Here is a great affirmation: "I accept and trust that what I need to heal this situation will now come to me."

Someone said, "You will be sick until you are sick of being sick." In other words, "You will get off it when you are *ready* to get off it." One day you decide this attention you enjoy from the illness is not worth it. Or you decide you have had enough of your excuses. Or you decide you no longer have any more fear of being in your full power. Or you finally forgive. Or whatever.

Many times, students who have already taken my spiritual healing class come to me and complain about some ailment they have had for a long time. I ask them, "Well, what did you get when you did the Ultimate Truth Process?" Then they confess to me that they did not even do it.

I ask, "Why not?"

"Oh, I forgot," they say.

I was always so surprised at this answer at first. But now I understand how tricky the ego is. It distracts you from what works. You must train yourself to do the Ultimate Truth Process as soon as you get the symptoms, so they won't escalate. Sometimes people "forget" because, as I already mentioned, they have a deep unconscious fear of going against the church that told them they must suffer. That distorts their thinking. In that case, the person needs to be helped by someone like me or someone else who is no longer trapped in that dogma.

13.

Finding the Solution

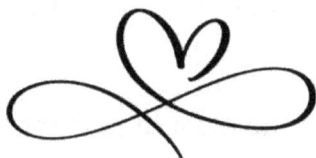

Important Points

1. The part of your mind that is *real*, that of the Holy Spirit's mind, is totally alive and perfect. It is *always* stronger than any mistaken thought of your ego. Your ego miscreated the negative condition. Say, "I am stronger than this _____." or "The God in me is stronger than _____."

Remember again that anything you have created, you can uncreate. It is *less work* to heal yourself than to make yourself sick. It takes effort and struggle to hang onto negative thinking to make yourself sick. Your natural state is health. You had to work at going against your natural state to have created this condition.

2. Anything on its way up is on its way *out*. That is another way of saying that your symptom is the cure in process. It is no longer suppressed!

3.You may need to get a Liberation Breathwork practitioner sooner than you think—one who knows how to "process" or clear your resistance to healing. The Breathworker should be able to help you get to the cause of the condition, help you breathe it out, and help you process it yourself. If the healing does not work, it is because you are blocking it.

The *will to live* is the most important factor in your healing. If your life urge is strong enough, you can overcome any condition. If you get stuck in fear or think, "I might die," you will weaken greatly and inhibit the natural healing abilities of the body. Recently I read an article about a man who had severe metastasis of cancer. He reversed it all and came out clean, much to the shock of doctors who could hardly accept his healing. The one thing I remember about the article is that he said he *never* entertained the thought that he was going to die. He was able to have absolute certainty – and it worked.

Faith is everything! When your faith is weak and the temptation to think that you won't make it takes over, that is exactly when you need to pray more, get Breathwork, and get spiritual support.

14.

Spiritual Background

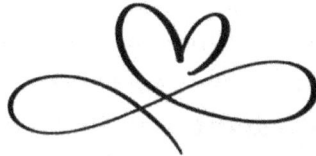

A Course in Miracles in Review

A Course in Miracles is a correction of religion. It is important to understand how false religious theology ruins and runs our lives. It is important to understand how it affects our minds, our bodies, and our health. Naturally, much of what we learned in church, mosque, or synagogue was wonderful; however, some teachings were intolerably confusing. Until those points are cleared up, it is hard to figure out permanent healing.

For example, the old church paradigm teaches that we are separate from God. This mistaken theology leads us to believe that we must die to be with God in heaven; therefore, we get sick and age. We think we are bad for being here because we "left" God to get here and that we are sinners of the worst kind. If we believe this, we will have tremendous guilt, and guilt demands punishment. One of the main ways we punish ourselves is by damaging our bodies, getting sick, aging, and finally choosing death as the final punishment. A Course calls this our descent into hell while here on earth.

The church teaches that heaven is somewhere else and is our goal. Therefore, we cannot really wait to leave here, and as a result, we are not fully here. The church also implies that somewhere else, like Heaven, is so much better that we are eager to leave the earth and get there. What nobody tells you is that consciousness seeks its own level when you drop your body. You are always going to have to face where you are no matter where you are. Furthermore, you are going to have to keep coming back here until you attain enlightenment and forgive everyone and everything. So, try to get enlightened asap while you are here now.

The church also implies that we should not have too much fun or joy while we are here. Therefore, the joy of permanent healing is something we think we do not deserve. Confusion reigns and leaves us tied up in knots. We learn that we are not allowed to question the church, or we might go to hell. How, then, can we get anything straight? This is exactly why we need A Course in Miracles—to straighten things out.

ACIM is not a religion or a *path*. It is a correction. When you read it, you will know it came from Jesus and there is only one appropriate response: gratitude to Him. The reason it is Christian in tone is because Christianity must be corrected first since it is such a major influence on the planet. No body of knowledge exists that does not need to be corrected and upgraded. However, many religions are threatened by the ideas in ACIM, because it challenges what is false. Some do not want to change even though they profess that they do not like the horrors afflicting society and that something must be done. Before anyone adversely criticizes ACIM, I should think they need to read it all the way through, and they would change their tune.

A Course in Miracles explains that everything we know is wrong, so we must start over. (Our results should show us that.) Everything is wrong because we interpret everything through the ego. The ego is a false self that we made up to compete with God. It is based on the erroneous thought, "I am separate from God." Once we believed that, we went into weakness, helplessness, fear, anxiety, suffering, anger, misery, sickness, aging, and death. The ego is a collection of all our negative thinking that keeps us from remembering we are one with God. Furthermore, the results of God are always Joy. So, if we are not supremely happy, then something is terribly off.

In the ego's interpretation, this separation is real and actually happened. Therefore, God is out to destroy us for this. We try to bargain with God, saying, "You don't have to go to the trouble of punishing me; I will punish myself." The idea of sacrifice was then formed: "I will suffer and deprive myself to prove I am good, so you won't be angry, God." In the ego's thought system, we get the insane notion that sacrifice is salvation, that God's will for us is perfect misery, and that we do not deserve to be happy. Furthermore, we think that the more we suffer now, the better off we will be later (such as in heaven).

The ego's version is that we must perish. (I acknowledge the great teacher Ken Wapnick, one of the leading experts on ACIM, for helping me understand the Course.)

The ego's interpretation of the crucifixion is that only one of God's sons (Jesus) had to suffer to free us all. This interpretation lays more guilt on our heads; that is, how does it make you feel if someone who is totally pure must die for you? This interpretation, Ken explained, does not make us feel free of guilt at all; it makes us feel MORE guilty. Yet salvation is supposed to free us from guilt. We do not really understand the crucifixion. A Course in Miracles explains that the crucifixion was an extreme teaching device. It shows that no perception of oneself as a victim is justified. It explains that Jesus did not defend himself, nor did he even believe he was attacked. He saw only threatened people who did not think they deserved the love of God.

In ACIM, Jesus says that the truth is that there is no sin because there is no separation. The truth is that it is impossible for us to be separate from God. Therefore, we are innocent. All sins are forgiven because they never really occurred. There is no need for sacrifice. Because we are innocent, we do not need to suffer, and because that is true, we can also give ourselves perfect health now!

Personally, it has taken me a long time to digest ACIM because I was addicted to the dogma of the church for so many lifetimes. I, like most people, brought to this life certain core beliefs that seemed impossible to change; beliefs such as "We are sinners." It seemed that if I gave up the thought that I am a sinner, I would *really* be a sinner. Or if I dared think I was innocent, I would *really* be guilty. This is the trap of the ego. What helped me most was to remember this: if there is a lie at the center of a thought system, the whole system is deceptive! Since the lie at the center of my religion was that one is separated from God, I had to admit that the whole religion is off. Even after I understood that I was still afraid because the church had an extra, built-in control: if I questioned or tried to leave, I would surely die and go to hell. That kept me stuck.

One day I realized all this was ridiculous because on one hand, they used the threat of death to control me, and on the other hand, they promoted death as something to look forward to for final peace! This double bind was not resolvable, and so I knew it had to be off. I resented being put into this trap my whole life. I regretted buying into it. Through prayer and help from my teachers, I have been able to unravel this conflict to the point that things make more sense. I know now that many of the illnesses I had manifested were a direct result of this religious brainwashing and confusion. (Some people now call it religious abuse.)

I am not on a campaign to attack religion. I have tried to forgive all false religious theology. What I want is to be able to understand what is false and what is real, and Jesus is telling us *how*. He says the Holy Spirit was placed in our minds as a solution to our imagined separation. To Jesus, our identity is Spirit. Therefore, we are love, joy, happiness, bliss, peace, and perfect health. There is even the possibility of immortality if one follows his words and practices spiritual laws. He said in the Bible: "If you follow me, you will never see the grave." Few could do it; however, some DID and became immortal masters who ascended (dematerialized).

Often when immortals try to explain that giving up the death urge is the key to having perfect health and that physical immortality is a real possibility, others cannot accept such information because their minds are in the other framework (ego). It is like talking to a wall or speaking in a foreign language. To understand the idea of permanent healing, one must have their mind in the opposite framework and know the difference between the ego's thought system and the Holy Spirit's thought system. (This is not Freud's definition of the ego.) People in the ego's thought system think that death is inevitable (and it will be). *They think death is the will of God.*

The problem is that the ego tries to keep us from learning that which would heal us. There may be tremendous resistance even to buying ACIM. There could be more resistance to reading it. The book says that ACIM is REQUIRED if you want to make it in life—only the time you take is voluntary. This means you can get it in the next five months, the next five years, or the next five lifetimes. WHY WAIT?

Below are selections from A Course in Miracles. Read them as many times as it takes for you to understand what is being said. It could be the key to your healing and health.

All sickness and symptoms are part of the death urge and ego. Sickness and death are correlative.

> *Death is not your Father's will nor yours. The death penalty is the ego's ultimate goal, for it truly believes that you are a criminal deserving death. The death penalty never leaves the ego's mind, for that is what it always reserves for you in the end. It will torment you while you live, but its hatred is not satisfied until you die. As long as you feel guilty, you are listening to the voice of the ego, which tells you that you have been treacherous to God and therefore deserve death.*
>
> *You will think that death comes from God and not from the ego, because confusing*

yourself with the ego, you think you want death. When you are tempted by the desire of death, remember that I DID NOT DIE. [Jesus speaking]. Would I have overcome death for myself alone? And would eternal life be given it to you?

When you learn to make ME [Jesus] manifest, you will never see death. God did not make death. But if you use the world for what is not its purpose, you will not escape the laws of disease, violence, and death. Forget not that the healing of God's sons (all souls) is all the world is for.

No one can die unless he chooses death. What seems to be the fear of death is really its attraction.

When you make sin real, you request death. To the ego, sin means death, so atonement is achieved through murder!

Death is the result of the thought we call the ego, just as surely as life is the result of the thought we call God.

Death is an attempt to resolve conflict by not deciding at all. Like any other solution the ego attempts, it will not work. To the ego, the goal is death. The ego is insane.

(Compiled from various passages from the Text of A Course in Miracles)

The cause of all pain and sickness is always the wish to die and conquer the Christ. This must be faced. (The ego is in competition with God. The ego causes sickness and pain.)

ACIM says hell is what the ego makes of the *present*. The way out of our own hell is to accept the Atonement for ourselves. That means inviting in the

Holy Spirit and accepting the correction of all our wrong thinking. It means not giving support of agreement to anyone else's illusions of sickness and death. It means having the right perception of the body.

> *When the body becomes an empty space, without any purpose other than the one the Holy Spirit gives it, it can become a sign of life, a promise of redemption, a breath of immortality to those grown sick of breathing in the fetid scent of death. The Will of God, who created neither sin nor death, wills that you not be bound by them.*

Jesus goes on to say in ACIM that nothing is accomplished through death. Everything is accomplished through life, and life is of the mind and in the mind. He says that if we share the same mind, we can overcome death, because He did.

The Importance of Forgiveness

❖ To hold a grievance is to let the ego rule and condemn the body to death.

❖ Holding a grievance is an attack on God's plan for salvation, and excludes yourself from salvation.

❖ Each grievance keeps you in darkness and will destroy the body.

❖ All healing is the result of some kind of forgiveness.

❖ Forgiveness is release. There is no pain or illness forgiveness cannot heal.

❖ Forgiveness ends all suffering and loss.

❖ Forgiveness overlooks all sin. It does not make it real.

❖ Forgiveness is the only road that leads out of disaster, past all suffering and away from death.

❖ Those who withhold forgiveness are binding themselves to illusions. Those who forgive have everything.

❖ Forgiveness returns the mind to the awareness of God.

❖ Forgiveness allows love to return to awareness.

❖ Forgiveness is how we recognize our innocence.

❖ Forgiveness is our function as the light of the world.

❖ It is your forgiveness that lets you recognize you are the light.

❖ All forgiveness is a gift you give yourself.

❖ Forgiveness will remove all sense of weakness strain, and fatigue from your mind.

❖ Forgiveness lifts darkness and entitles you to vision.

❖ Forgiveness is the way Christ's vision comes to us. It is the means by which the mind returns to God.

❖ Only forgiveness sets us free. Only forgiveness restores peace.

❖ Salvation and forgiveness are the same.

In Lesson #122 of ACIM, the Christ Consciousness establishes these "Gifts of God:"

1. Do you want peace? Forgiveness offers it.
2. Do you want happiness? Forgiveness offers it.
3. Do you want a quiet mind? Forgiveness offers it.
4. Do you want a certainty of purpose? Forgiveness offers it.
5. Do you want a sense of worth and beauty that transcends the world? Forgiveness offers it.
6. Do you want care? Forgiveness offers it.
7. Do you want safety? Forgiveness offers it.
8. Do you want the warmth of sure protection always? Forgiveness offers it.
9. Do you want a quietness that cannot be disturbed? Forgiveness offers it.
10. Do you want a gentleness that never can be hurt? Forgiveness offers it.
11. Do you want deep abiding comfort and health? Forgiveness offers it.
12. Do you want a rest so perfect it can never be upset? Forgiveness offers it.

The purpose of A Course in Miracles is the escape from fear

(From Lesson #190 in ACIM)
Read the following out loud to yourself.

"Pain is a sign illusions rule in place of the truth. It demonstrates God is denied, confused with fear, perceived as mad, and seen as traitor to himself. If God is real, there is no pain. If pain is real, there is no God. Fear, denying love and using pain to prove that God is dead, has shown that death is victor over life. Pain is the thought of evil taking form and working havoc in your holy mind."

Now read the above again, substituting sickness for the word pain.

"All forms of sickness, even unto death are physical expressions of fear of awakening. Healing is the release from fear of waking. Sinlessness is the escape from fear." (Chapter 8 of Text of ACIM)

"Death is the symbol of the fear of God. God did not make death because he did not make fear."
(ACIM: Manual for Teachers)

"The unforgiving mind is full of fear."
(ACIM: Workbook; Lesson #121)

"What is not love is always fear."
(ACIM: Text; from Chapter 15)

Below is continuation of my personal notes from ACIM from an old notebook I ran across recently taken in the late 1970s.

Notes from class on A Course in Miracles

I found an old notebook of mine which contained notes from classes by my teacher Ken Wapnick. I wrote them down back in the 1970's in San Francisco. I recommend all his books.

Some of these notes are things already mentioned in this book but some are not. Anyway, it never hurts to hear some statements over and over.

Notes:

Healing occurs when the valuelessness of sickness is recognized. One must but say this: "There is no gain at all to me in this."

If the patient uses sickness as a way of life, sudden healing might precipitate intense depression. Healing will then wait. The instant it is welcome, it is there.

Oneness and sickness cannot co-exist. One who has peacefully accepted the Atonement for himself has overcome death because he has accepted life. There is then no limit to his power of healing.

There is no problem the Holy Spirit cannot solve by offering you a miracle. (Of course, you would have to give up your addiction to the problem and you would have to be free of your fear of the miracle.)

Say this: "I accept the Holy Spirit's purpose for my body. It is not a scapegoat for my guilt. **My body is for the word of God.**"

Miracles cannot be performed in a state of fear or doubt. Ask for help to clear the conditions that brought about the fear.

Atonement = Perfect Love & awareness that the separation never really occurred. The Atonement heals with certainty. It takes away the guilt.

All healing is release from the past. However, the ego cannot tolerate release from the past. So one has to invite in the Holy Spirit for this to happen.

The guiltless mind cannot suffer. The continuing decision to remain separated is the only possible reason for continuing guilt feelings. One has to pray for release of the addiction to guilt.

ALL SALVATION is the escape from guilt.

Had you not lacked faith that your problem could be solved, it would be gone. **There is no problem in any situation that faith will not solve.** Ask to have your faith restored where it was lost.

One must want the HOLY INSTANT above all else...and one must know that one is worthy of it. Accepting it is reaching another state of mind where the answer is.

The glitter of guilt you laid upon your body would kill you. **No one can die unless he chooses death.** God, who created neither sin nor death wills not that you be bound by them. The belief in sin is the request for death.

Everything that seems to happen to you, you asked for it. (Unconsciously.) It is impossible that happenings that come to you were never your choice.

Your power of decision is the determining factor in every situation you find yourself, by chance or accident.

The healing of God's Son is all the world is for. If you use it for any other purpose, you will not escape the laws of violence and death.

Death is the opposite of peace because it is the opposite of life. Life is peace. To hold a grievance is to let the ego rule and condemn the body to death.

Death takes on many forms. **It may appear as sadness, fear, anxiety, anger, faithlessness, lack of trust, envy, and concern for bodies.** (All these things are due to what we call the Unconscious Death Urge.)

Pain demonstrates God is denied, confused with fear, and perceived as mad.

Swear not to die, you holy son of God. You were not born to die. **Life's function cannot be to die.**

The only thing that is required for healing is a lack of fear.

Sickness is anger taken out onto the body so it will suffer pain.

A sick body does not make any sense because it is not what the body is for. That is based on the idea that the body is for attack.

The sick remain accusers. They cannot forgive their brothers or themselves.

If you believe you can be sick, you have placed other gods before Him. **That's why sickness is blasphemy.**

You can be hurt by nothing but your thoughts and you can elect to change all thoughts that hurt.

If you think one thing is harder to heal than another, then you don't think everything is one and you are denying God His ability to bestow His blessing of healing onto you.

It is a "power trip" to not let anyone heal you and you do this number because **you are in competition with God and you want to be "king."**

You deserve to be released from the Hell you made. But the Holy Spirit cannot take from you your defects without your willingness because that would violate free will.

Each time you keep a problem for yourself to solve, or judge that it is one that has no resolution, **you have made it great and past the hope of healing.**

The ego tricks you into thinking that surrender is weakness.

Since you believe that you are separate, Heaven consciousness seems separate too. **Heaven is a decision you must make.** Heaven is the state of perfect Oneness.

If God is just, there can be no problem that justice cannot solve.

If you know that you are One with God, no miracle can be denied.

You will receive whatever you request. All you need to do is to wish Heaven be given to you instead of Hell.

The outcome of your condition is what you decide. There is nothing you cannot do.

15.

The Holy Instant

(A Chapter by Markus Ray)

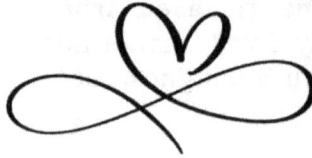

The Holy Instant is a moment in time in which time is actually suspended. One could accurately call it a "moment outside of time." This also means that memory is suspended. It possesses qualities not like anything that came before.

There were moments I had with my teacher, Tara Singh, that were clearly Holy Instants. In fact, my whole purpose in knowing him was an action of Life that was giving me these experiences. I received them not because of wanting them, or from a deep-seeded need to understand them, although I did read in A Course in Miracles that they were possible. I received them out of Grace. Pure and simple—God's Grace bestowed them upon me, just as God's Grace had put me together with my teacher, Tara Singh.

I have written extensively about my relationship with Tara Singh in two of my books, *Miracles with My Master, Tara Singh,* and *The Master Is Beautiful.* I need not reiterate here the importance of having a Spiritual Master in one's life—a person who can guide us through the tougher lessons of an ascension process that would open us up to experiencing these "Holy Instants."

The Holy Instant refers to one's choice to accept the energy of love over fear, and unity over separation. It may require a lifetime of practice. Around A Holy Instant are often the conditions that would bring up the most fear in us, and compel us to withdraw and isolate ourselves, rather than join and unify. This is why a teacher is needed to help us break through these difficult conditions.

A Spiritual Master helps us to *surrender*. This element of *letting go* is absolutely essential to having the Holy Instant. A Course in Miracles refers a lot to the Holy Instant. There is a whole Chapter 15 in the Text that is dedicated to the Holy Instant. It starts by saying this:

> *Can you imagine what it means to have no cares, no worries, no anxieties, but merely to be perfectly calm and quiet all the time? Yet that is what time is for; to learn just that and nothing more. God's Teacher cannot be satisfied with His teaching until it constitutes all your learning. He has not fulfilled His teaching function until you have become such a consistent learner that you learn only of Him. When this has happened, you will no longer need a teacher or time in which to learn. (ACIM; Text; Chapter 15; Section I; ¶1)*

"God's Teacher" is ultimately the Christ. The Christ is a consciousness that was made manifest in the man Jesus, but it is an awareness of oneness so complete that it can be extended to those whom He touches.

One could say Krishna had Christ Consciousness; Babaji had it. The Buddha as well. Any Spiritual Master, man or woman, has Christ Consciousness, not just Jesus. For me, this touch upon my shoulder came in the form of Tara Singh, who was making the Christ Consciousness manifest in my life. Naturally I would feel and have these Holy Instants around him, more than with any other person in my life up until the time of our meeting. He had received many Holy Instants from his teachers, Mr. Krishnamurti and Dr. Helen Schucman, so he was well versed in receiving and giving them by the time we met in March of 1989, Easter weekend.

"I have nothing to teach. You know too much already." These were the first words I heard my teacher utter to me in person. That was the first Holy Instant I had with Tara Singh. The implication was that the things I had "learned" were actually blocks in my awakening process. I had learned a lot of negative thoughts that were not part of my Divine makeup, and in order to make contact with my Holy Nature, these would have to be undone, removed, and forgiven. This was a process into which I entered with Tara Singh for the next seventeen years of my life. At the time I did not know the length of this Holy Relationship, that goes on even to this day.

In the Holy Instant our thought does not mean anything. For an instant we are free of it. What are we using then, in this space free of thought?

God's Thought may not need words to express It. It is an energy of deep well-being. An energy of stillness permeates this inner peace and joy. Our own thought is silenced, and from these *sounds* we hear without the body's ears, and *sights* we see without the body's eyes, we are cleansed and made whole. We share in a remarkable sense of Oneness. No separation divides us into parts, nor defines us in terms of a personality we made up. We are disassociated from the little "self" we made up, and totally immersed in the Greater Self God Created.

We make contact with our Christ Self, shared not only with our brother, or teacher in my case, but with the rest of Creation Itself. We essentially witness the end of separation and feel the Love of God within us, if only for an instant. We feel that connection with every atom in the universe. There is no sense of separation. We are in a stillness and silence so profound there is no place or time we would rather be than "now."

Later, A Course in Miracles teaches, "This instant is the only time there is." (ACIM; Workbook; Lesson #308)

> *The only interval in which I can be saved from time is now. For in this instant has forgiveness come to set me free. The birth of Christ is now, without a past or future. He has come to give His present blessing to the world, restoring it to timelessness and love. And love is ever-present, here and now.*

Taraji used to tell us, "Peace is always here, but you are absent." Meaning, whatever strife and struggle we are experiencing, we are making that up ourself, because we are unwilling to be in the frequency of the Peace that is here now. Once this is pointed out, and some degree of surrender takes place in us, we are able to make this contact with the actuality of our Holiness. This contact we could say is a Holy Instant.

Being with a person like Tara Singh, who was always in the present with the Peace of God, had an impact on me. When I was with him, the Holy Instant was not only present, but it was extended into all of the time I spent with him. Being with Tara Singh was like being in "consecutive moments of now." And that "now" was the most sacred space I could have ever imagined. The stillness and the silence of it contributed to an inner peace, and a sense of beauty and grace that transcended the world, the likes of which I had never known.

The Holy Instant is nothing short of an actual contact with the Holy Spirit, and with this contact comes certainty. The Holy Spirit is the communication link between God and us, while we are still being fooled in our separated state. It is God's gift and is the voice for God. It is the mechanism for miracles. It is the mediator between illusions and the truth. It is the bringer of the Holy Instant in our life. We need to nurture a relationship with the Holy Spirit—an energy of undoing the false in us, that can make the conditions perfect to receive the true in us. My time with Tara Singh had its challenges, mostly on my part, to let go of enough of my ego in order to meet him in the present, free of my illusions.

When I was willing to do that in the most sincere and humble way, the miraculous unfolded in my life, and I experienced with him these many moments of perfect peace. This is the purpose of the real teacher and student relationship—it is a Holy encounter in which the Truth of Oneness is shared— a Holy Instant.

16.

Physical Immortality

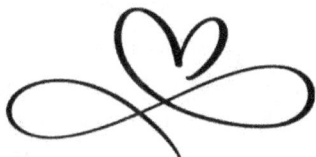

If you can destroy your body, you can just as well preserve it. However, if you believe death is inevitable and that you are separate from God, you are in the process of dying right now.

"Oh," you might say, "a hundred years of this is all I can take." This statement springs from a deep-rooted belief in suffering and limitation. You have not yet experienced the fullness of health, joy, wisdom, peace, and love. You are given how to have these substantive qualities of life itself; and once you have them, why leave?

The corollary of death is sickness. A Course in Miracles says that sickness is idolatry!

Some people say, "Well, I am willing to live forever if it does not get too bad." That is a cop-out because it only gets too bad if one has not given up loyalty to death. In other words, the reason one has pain, suffering, misery, and a bad time is precisely because of hanging onto the death urge.

People think they age, get sick, and die. The truth is that you die in your mind, you get sick, and then you age. You create symptoms in your body that make it socially acceptable to leave it.

Your beliefs (thoughts you keep thinking) control your physical body. If you think you are going to die, you will. However, death is *optional.* And there is an alternative to aging! The key is to stop affirming that "death is inevitable." Remember instead what Lessons #162 & #163 in A Course in Miracles say: "I am as God created me." And "There is no death, the Son of God is free." And further on it says that, "He who lives by these words will never look upon death." When you choose these thoughts instead of affirming death, your health will improve.

Choosing life strengthens your body the most. That means choosing life so fully that you love it so much you want to live forever. That kind of passion is what works! Physical immortality can be defined as "endless existence," specifically the endless existence of your physical body in perpetual health and youthfulness. The body may look different; it would be a "diamond body." The diamond body is discussed later in this chapter.

We are not talking about living in an old body for hundreds of years; we are talking about learning to rejuvenate the body and reverse the aging process. Your body can produce new cells. (You have seen this many times; for example, when you repair a cut.) Your body is a constantly flowing stream of life. It has a built-in regeneration battery. If you use your mind correctly, you are in charge of how you flow your stream of life.

If you are tempted by the idea that you are not one with God (and cannot determine the consequences of your own actions) and are not in charge of your own body, it is all over. Once you invalidate your divinity in this manner and think you are a sinner, you will give in to helplessness and think, "I cannot heal myself," or "I am weak," or "God is going to destroy me since I am so bad."

Spiritual masters do not think like that. They remember who they are. That is the difference. Some can rapidly youth or age their bodies at will, and some can even transform into male or female, a child, or an elderly person at will. Babaji is an example of such a master. (Read Chapters 33 & 34 in *The Autobiography of a Yogi* by Paramahansa Yogananda and our book *Babaji: My Miraculous Meetings with a Maha Avatar.* bit.ly/BabajiRay)

God is not only love, but God is *life;* life without beginning or end. God is not the author of anything that is not Himself. In the Book of Ezekiel, we are told that He wills *not* the death of any, but that all should turn to Him and *live.*

The body is the temple of the living God. But remember this: It is possible to weaken the soul's hold on the body with the thought that death is inevitable or with the thought that disease is stronger than the power of God. Don't ever allow yourself to think that any disease is stronger than the power of God! This is a departure from Divine Mind and is based on a subtle misconception about the purpose of life and the significance of the body.

The Bible presents death as the last enemy to be destroyed. Revelation 21:4 says, "And God shall wipe away all tears and there shall be no more death."

The reason for living a long time would never be so that you could brag you are 150 years old! The reason would be because you are on a mission of Divine Service.

All healing is temporary until you heal death. We could teach you how to heal cancer (cancer is a battle between the life urge and the death urge and the cells are confused). But if you do not heal your death urge, you will just make up a new way to kill yourself!

Affirmations

- ❖ I am alive now, therefore my life urges are stronger than my death urges. As long as I continue strengthening my life urges and weakening my death urges, I will go on living in health and youthfulness.
- ❖ Life is eternal and I am life. My mind, as the thinking quality of life itself, is eternal. My physical body is also eternal if I say so. Therefore, my living flesh has a natural tendency to live forever in perfect health and youthfulness.
- ❖ My physical body is a safe and pleasurable place for me to be. The entire universe exists for the purpose of supporting my physical body and for providing a pleasurable place for me to express myself.
- ❖ All the cells of my body are daily bathed in the perfection of my divine being.
- ❖ The more I am good to myself, the more I enrich my own aliveness.

The Last Initiation

The last initiation has to do with the physical body, our "last burden." Let's look closer at what is meant by the transformation of the physical organism. Earlier reference was made to the "diamond body," and the next several paragraphs from *Being, Evolution, and Immortality* by Hindu Scholar Haridas Chaudhuri clarify this concept of transformation.

> *Finally, the concept of immortality implies a harmonization of the entire personality and a transformation of the physical organism as an effective channel of expression of higher values. This may be called material immortality.*
>
> *There are some mystics and spiritual seekers who strengthen and purify their bodies just enough to be able to experience the thrilling touch of the Divine. They use the body as a ladder—climbing toward a pure spiritual level. On attaining that level, the body is felt as a burden, as a prison house, as a string of chains that holds one in bondage. Dissociation from this "last burden" of the body is considered a sine qua non for total liberation. Continued association with the body is believed to be the result of the residual trace of ignorance.*
>
> *The body is not only a ladder that leads to the realm of immortality of the soul, but it is also an excellent instrument for expressing the glory of physical immortality in life and society. It is capable of being thoroughly penetrated by the light of the Spirit. It is capable of being transformed into what has been called the "diamond body." As a result of such*

transformation, the body does not appear anymore to be a burden on the liberated self. It shines as the Spirit made flesh. It functions as a very effective instrument for creative action and realization of high values in the world. It is purged of all inner tension and conflict. It is liberated from the anxiety of repressed wishes. It is also liberated from the dangerous grip of the death impulse born of self-repression. Mystics who look on the body as a burden suffer from anxiety of self-repression and the allurement of the death wish.

Material immortality means decisive victory over both these demons. It conquers the latent death instinct in man and fortifies the will to live as long as is necessary as a channel of expression of the Divine. It also liquidates all forms of self-suppression, self-torture, and self-mutilation. As a result, the total being of an individual becomes strong and steady, whole, and healthy. There is a meaningful self-expression. Under the guidance of the indwelling light of the Eternal, it produces increasing manifestations of the spirit in matter.

Lesson #163 in ACIM talks about how we are the ones that make death inevitable. Here is the first paragraph of the lesson: "There is no death. The Son of God is free. Death is a thought that takes on many forms, often unrecognized. It may appear as sadness, fear, anxiety, or doubt; as anger, faithlessness and lack of trust, concern for bodies, envy, and all forms in which the wish to be as you are not may come to tempt you. All such thoughts are but reflections of the worshipping of death as savior, and as giver of release. God made not death."

"When your forgiveness lessons are complete, then not one trace of guilt will remain in your unconscious mind. At that point, you will break the cycle of birth and death, and never dream of reincarnating." (*Your Immortal Reality* by Gary Renard)

The Manual for Teachers of A Course in Miracles in Section 12 gives us the final word on the final initiation. "The central lesson is always this: that what you use the body for it will become to you. Use it for attack, which is the same as sin, and you will see it as sinful. Because it is sinful it is weak and being weak it suffers and dies. Use it to bring the word of God to those who have it not, and the body becomes holy. Because it is holy it cannot be sick, nor can it die. When its usefulness is done it is laid by and that is all. The mind makes this decision, as it makes all decisions that are responsible for the body's condition."

Life and death are functions of consciousness. If we believe "death is inevitable" then our consciousness is filled with the "shelf-life" concept that brings about entropy. If we are willing to question this thought, we open up to a new possibility. At least we see that life and death are matters that *we decide*, not matters that *decide for us*. We rule our minds in all cases, even on this subject, and we can affect the outcome of how we live, and for how long, with the power of our own Divine Mind.

17.

Happiness Equals Health

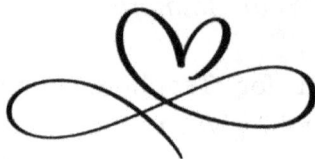

Many people think or say, "I won't be happy until I am healthy." This is understandable, yet the truth is that you will be healthy when you are happy. If you read Deepak Chopra's books, especially *Quantum Healing*, this becomes very clear; he explains it scientifically. He also makes clear that unhappiness is due to loss of contact with the Source, which means that people forget that they are one with God.

Mother Teresa said that most people are spiritually deprived, and that is the whole problem with the world. This is very important, yet when people are told to become spiritual to be happy, they often rebel. They are likely to think that means they must go back to something such as the church or some kind of dogma. They usually do not want to do so, because they have rarely seen it work for their parents and/or they have been disappointed in religion themselves.

Becoming more spiritual is really finding the deeper Self that is *real*—that self that possesses absolute wisdom and self-knowledge. Dr. Chopra says that in India, finding the "knower" is considered life's greatest adventure. That is exactly why I love to go to India each year! I cherish having the opportunity to be with the great saints who are bursting with joy. In one's spiritual life, this is called the "principle of right association"—placing oneself with the highest beings possible so that one is forced to adapt *upward!*

Robert Johnson, in his book *Transformation: Understanding the Three Levels of Masculine Consciousness* writes: "Happiness derives from the verb *to happen.* Happiness is to be found simply from observing what happens. If you cannot be happy at the prospect of lunch, you are not likely to find happiness anywhere. What happens is happiness."

The idea, of course, is to be happy no matter what goes on around you *and* to know how to be happy without your happiness depending on material things. You must also remember that all misery is self-inflicted and that blaming the world for unhappy situations will never work. All this has to do with handling your mind. Your mind-body system must be connected with pure consciousness. (In transcendental meditation, it is called the "unified field," which is the source of all energy fields and fundamental particles.) ACIM refers to this as the Holy Spirit. When we are then aware of our connection to that, as Dr. Chopra says, all existence is experienced once again as bliss.

"Bliss," Maharishi, the founder of transcendental meditation, says, "is ultimately the most powerful agent of physiology." Maharishi says that "any attempt to treat disease or any form of suffering on the physical level is too superficial. Bliss is the fundamental nature of the Self." The method that Maharishi and Deepak Chopra recommend for experiencing the state of bliss is to settle the mind through transcendental meditation. We use Liberation Breathing to achieve happiness. It is a breathing meditation. It is a "silencing of the mind of thought," to enter into the pure stillness of the soul.

In my book *Pure Joy*, I list many other methods of spiritual purification that help you return to that state of bliss. Arranging your life so you are happy about your surroundings, your job, your relationships, and your situations is important, but not nearly as important as the state of your mind. You may be in a job and/or a relationship that is not right for you, which is not a good idea. I know many people who stay in dead or destructive relationships because they are afraid to leave. Staying in a relationship you do not want to be in just because you are afraid to leave and/or afraid to be alone is not a good reason to be there. Is it even ethical? (You CAN create a new relationship easily by the power of your mind.) *Spiritual Intimacy* occurs when two people are clear that they come together for the evolution of their souls. This includes spiritual purification that helps each partner ascend the ladder of holiness, which is being in a state of mind that results in perfect happiness.

Staying in a job that makes you unhappy does not make any sense either. If you do not like the way things are in your life, change them! You may have to leave your job, your marriage, your area, or whatever. It may be just your attitude, however, and even if you change all these external things but do not change your attitude, the same thing could come up elsewhere. First try loving where you are, whom you are with, and what you are doing, and see what happens. If you are unhappy in your relationship, maybe you just need to take our Loving Relationships Training (The LRT®).

Many people are unhappy because they have no idea why they are here or what their purpose of life is. Nothing really "hangs together" for them. I could say a lot on this subject, but let's get clear on one thing: the purpose of life is not just to get married, have children, and then die. The purpose of life is to recognize the Supreme (according to my teacher Shastriji). The Supreme is Pure Joy. This means that you really need to think about your priorities. Are you, for example on the spiritual path of becoming all that you can be? Supremely happy all of the time?

The formula for happiness from my guru Babaji is this: Truth, Simplicity, Love, and Service to mankind. (He also recommends the mantra "Om Namaha Shivay" for purity.) Do you understand that all work is worship and that you should dedicate it to God daily? This changes everything.

Readiness and willingness to do any work at any time in any circumstance is the hallmark of spirituality. Spiritual people do it with love and sincerity, without expecting anything. That is why there is always charm and beauty in whatever spiritual people do. They love to do the work because the work itself gives them infinite happiness. When one worries about the result, the work loses its beauty.

> *To derive the full benefit of any action, whatever it may be, love for that particular action is absolutely necessary.* Mata Amritanandamayi, *Awaken Children* (p. 260)

This may be great, you might say, but you feel really, really depressed and cannot relate to any of this. What about depression? Depression can be understood like any other symptom and treated spiritually. Find its cause using the Ultimate Truth Process in this book. (Chapter #20.) Then start Liberation Breathing! A Course in Miracles says that all depression (like sickness) is an *idol* that is made up as a substitute for God!

We have found in Breathwork that the main cause of depression is the unconscious death urge. As I said earlier, this is a "consciousness factor" that includes your programming on death, the thought that death is inevitable, your secret wish to die because you hate your life, past-life memories of dying, the thought "I am separate from God," and other anti-life thoughts. All of that can surely make a person depressed!

My very first client as a Breathworker was a real test for me. She came to me very depressed, saying she wanted to kill herself. She was suicidal and said she did NOT want me to talk her out of it. She went on and on about why she wanted to die. I listened but knew that the part of her that wanted to live had come to me for Breathwork. If she truly wanted to die, she would not have come, so I focused on THAT part of her mind. I honored her wish not to push her to live. I just asked her to lie down, breathe, and to postpone suicide for five days until her next Breathwork session. I checked on her every day. I did the same each session, asking her to postpone her suicide. After about eight sessions, she wanted to live! She had breathed out enough death urge in the sessions that she felt different. She later became a dancer and now is also happily married.

Even if you have a fatal illness and a bad prognosis, let me repeat what a teacher of mine said: "As long as you have one breath left, there is still a chance." He reminded us that Jesus took it even further and brought people back *after* they died. For more information on these kinds of cases, read *The Romeo Error* by Lyall Watson. Never give up!

You might say, "Right, okay, I have decided that I do not want to lead a boring life, have a boring job, have a boring relationship, or ruin my body but how am I guaranteed to get out of these dreary messes?"

Well, let's look at the boring mind aspect that goes before these results. Here is a statement from the founder of Rebirthing: "Most people fear eternal life more than they do physical death; but what they really fear is not eternal life of their bodies, but the eternal life of their boring minds! The essential characteristic of a boring person is the morbidity of the deathist mentality. Conquering death is the basic intelligence test of spiritual enlightenment. Remember: A deathist mentality is unhealthy for human beings." —Leonard Orr

Some will say, Leonard Orr left his body at 81 years old in 2019, so he did not "make it." But he laid the groundwork to reconsider this topic of life extension and breaking the death "habit." Brilliant geniuses in history often posited great advancements, such as Leonardo and the possibility of human flight. It was nearly another 400 years later that the Wright brothers were successful in human flight at Kitty Hawk. One could argue Leonardo did not "make it." But on the shoulders of his aspirations and ideas, a determined humanity finally did realize in the 20th century the actualization of his 15th century theories.

18.

Influence of Relationships

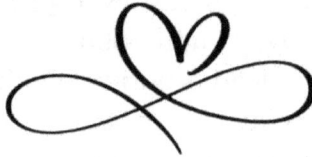

Negative relationships undermine health. The distress of that affects your immune system and the ability to heal. Distress in a relationship adversely affects our immune and hormonal systems.

Loneliness also has a bad effect on health. Loneliness is now considered as bad for your health as smoking!

A relationship can heal you or damage you more, depending on how you play the game of relationships.

You may want your mate to agree with you on everything and back you up no matter what. Or as a mate, you may think you are required to agree with him or her and back them up no matter what. This might look like a healed relationship, but what if it is just collusion and codependency that you are creating? In other words, what if your mate agrees with you just to make you happy, and what if you are into your ego or "case" at the time? He or she would be supporting your "case," supporting your ego, supporting that which will eventually make you sick and destroy you! When someone agrees with your case (your negative issues), how will that help you and heal you? It won't! Rather it will reinforce what you are supposed to be getting rid of. If you reinforce your case with the help of your mate, this will make it *more stuck,* and you have the likelihood of getting *sicker.*

The same is true vice versa—colluding with your mate could make her or him sicker. In the book *Love Without Conditions: Reflections of the Christ Mind,* my friend Paul Ferrini calls this "the tyranny of agreement." The ego cannot conceive that there is any love when two people disagree. If you support behavior that could be hurtful to your mate, this is the ultimate co-dependency. Peace does not come through the agreement of two egos. The truly healthy relationship has room for disagreement. YOU CAN EVEN DISAGREE WIHTOUT UPSETS! If you listen carefully to a mate who disagrees, you can learn what you need to change to stay healthy. Or, you become stronger in your convictions if they are truly founded.

Married couples often tend to think they must back their spouses no matter what. But what if your spouse is out of integrity? Does this mean you just TOLERATE your mate's issues? No. Rather than attack each other for issues or constantly disapprove of them, there is another approach. You and your mate have an agreement to help each other solve personal issues. Markus always has my permission to help me with my "case" and vice versa. The miracle we have is this: We are both Breathworkers so we can give each other sessions. We also each have sessions with other Breathworkers we respect to clear our issues. We try to never dump our issues on each other. I don't want to be sick, and I don't want him to get sick. He does not want to be sick, and he does not want me to be sick. We are very devoted to preventing illness by working on ourselves and we are both 100% committed to our enlightenment.

I have known married couples whom I also knew as single people before they met each other. Before meeting, they were each strong, with tremendous potential, often making great contributions. After moving in with each other, they more or less "caved in" on each other and became dependent and weak. They sold out, gave up dreams, and fell short of becoming all they could have been. I have often seen them almost destroy each other. Why?

A relationship should strengthen you, not weaken you. You should be happier because of the relationship, not more miserable. You should expand because of the relationship, not contract. You should get financially more prosperous, not less. You should get healthier, not sicker. This is the goal—the ideal. However, to handle everything that comes up in a relationship and to keep growing stronger, enlightenment is required. Instead of saying it feels impossible, study A Course in Miracles and see why the above is not happening for you. Read books on relationships, ours included.

If your mate becomes ill, your way of handling the condition also affects the outcome. If you both go into agreement with the illness, make it real, and give it undue attention, you are both reinforcing it. If you feel pity for your mate and treat them like an invalid, you make it worse. That does not mean you must be cold and ignore someone who needs support. The support he or she needs may not be what you thought. Encouragement and love without making someone more helpless is a good start!

See the person as healed. Envision them without the condition and help them heal by using the techniques in this book. Your confidence in a miraculous outcome can make a huge difference. I understand it is hard when you are in love with someone and you panic, thinking he or she might abandon you by being seriously ill or dying. You may need help yourself to hold the highest thought.

One of the best ways to support someone who has become ill is to help them remember to do the Ultimate Truth Process as soon as the symptoms surface. Do not wait until your mate gets a full-blown illness with a major diagnosis. Also study the ACIM supplements that explain how Jesus healed people. Try to align with His mind.

Many people stay in destructive or dead relationships because they are afraid to leave. This is not a good reason to stay, nor is it ethical. If you are lying to yourself and being unethical by staying, your chances for getting sick are greater.

People often ask me if they should leave a relationship immediately or wait and see if it ever clears up. This is not for me to decide. I tell them to pray for this relationship to be healed or for something better for both. Then, either way it is a win. I tell them to pray for divine right action. There are cases in which conditions suddenly shift and miracles happen, but we all know of cases in which people stayed too long and regretted it. Another thing I always ask is this: "If you had no fear and no guilt and you did not care what anyone said and if you knew you could create a new relationship, would you then stay or leave?" If they say, "I would leave," then I tell them they are out of integrity for staying. Staying because of fear is not ethical. If they say, "I would stay," well then, I can help them re-conceive the relationship.

The other day I heard from a woman who said, "It is strange how I had been hanging on to this extremely painful relationship and now I feel so *relieved* that it is over. I am like a new person." (I know if I had stayed in my first marriage, I would likely be sick right now and there would have been none of the trainings I wrote and led.)

Relationships are an integral part of inner healing. If your relationship is positive and supportive, healing will obviously happen faster. Make sure you are not in a relationship that inflicts further damage or despair. Make sure you are in a relationship that lifts you up, that gives you confidence and motivation. Also, make sure you are not around other people who bring you down.

Simply holding the hand of a loving partner can profoundly affect one greatly. It literally calms jittery neurons in the brain.

A happy, loving relationship is the goal, and the best way to have a perfect relationship is for both people to be willing to experience their own perfection. Commitment to self-improvement and spiritual enlightenment must be the top priority for both for the healing of the relationship to happen. Denying and pretending will only be destructive to the body.

Here is my suggestion.

Read our following 3 books for very helpful information on relationships:

I Deserve Love
bit.ly/DeserveRay

The New Loving Relationships Book
bit.ly/NLRBRay

Spiritual Intimacy
bit.ly/IntimacyRay

Also, we highly recommend you take the Loving Relationships Training (The LRT®).

19.

Influence of Communication

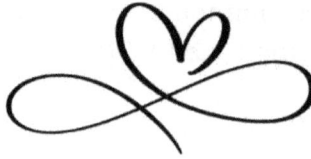

What you do *not* say could make you sick or keep you in pain. One of my early teachers, Werner Erhard, the founder of Erhard Seminars Training (EST), said, "What you cannot communicate runs you."

Some relationships have been destroyed because the couple never learned good communication habits. There is a vast improvement area in this for all of us. It is worth spending the time to study effective communication. Remember this: anger provokes separation. Communication ends separation. It is healing to be able to have great communication with someone. People feel better by being able to share. People just want to be heard. Maybe you are sick or in pain because you are afraid to say something to your mate.

I have heard of several cases in which people finally began communicating to a family member on her or his deathbed! The feeling may have been, "Well, since he is going to die anyway, saying this cannot kill him." I know a man who finally told his mother as she lay dying about something she had done that really bothered him. She was so sorry he had not told her sooner because the whole thing was a complete misunderstanding, a communication problem. She had meant just the opposite of the way he took it. The incident had negatively affected his life for nearly 40 years. Problems start from poor communication. Good communication will clear them up.

Years ago, a man in a group in San Diego studying communication developed what he called "compassionate communication." He recommended that a person say the following to their mate:

1. "What I observe in our relationship is . . ."
2. "What I feel about this is . . ."
3. "What I need and or recommend is . . ."

There is no blame or attack in this method. For example, instead of saying, "You don't handle this issue about the children. You never deal with it at all. You avoid everything. I don't think you are a good father, and you don't support me!" you would say:

- "What I notice is we are in conflict about (state the exact issue) bringing up the children."
- "What I feel is disappointed and anxious that we have not tried to resolve this issue together."
- "What I would like is for us to support each other and agree upon a resolution that is best for the children."

It is important to hear out everyone in a family and relationship. Give them space to say everything without interruption. Then say thank you instead of being on the defensive. This discharges the energy, and they will be able to drop the upset. You will be surprised at how much better you will feel physically after this simple procedure.

Markus and I came up with what we call "The Eight-Minute Communication Process." It goes like this:

A. If there are delicate things to discuss that could cause an argument, we recommend you go out for the discussion to a beautiful place such as a nice restaurant in a hotel. That is because there will usually be a carpet on the floor and soft music. These two things are important. If you go to an ordinary restaurant, chances are it will be noisy and there will be loud music. That will not do.

B. The person who is the most upset speaks first and is allowed to speak for eight minutes straight. (Set a timer.) The person speaking should use non-violent communication, no sentences beginning with "you," and no blame.

During those eight minutes, the listener obeys the following rules:

1. Absolutely no interruptions.
2. Listen to what is being said without rehearsing rebuttals.
3. Do not frown or make faces.
4. Keep eye contact, be caring, and sincerely try to understand what is being said.

C. After eight minutes, switch. This partner then shares what is on their mind, and whatever they feel is going on with themselves. It is not about commenting on what the other said as in a debate. It could be on any topic introduced by the person now speaking. It could be on the same topic, or it could be on a different topic.

D. After each person has spoken for eight minutes, there can be a healthy discussion; however, each must agree to continue to use compassionate and non-violent communication for the duration.

Another good thing to remember is that when a person is upset, it is best to listen and see if you can find one thing upon which you agree. You might not agree with much, but begin by saying, "I can see your point about ..." or "I agree with ..." Then stop to integrate this alignment.

Another thing to remember when you want to bring up something to a mate is to try to avoid a "harsh startup." That would be when you begin a conversation with blame. Avoid starting sentences with "You did _____," because that sounds like blame. A "soft startup" always helps. That would be when you begin a topic by pointing out your own part in any problem going on in the relationship.

Read the book *You Just Don't Understand* by Deborah Tannen to learn more about the differences in male and female communication.

The main point is that suppressing stuff hurts your body and leads to disease. Expressing things responsibly helps you stay healthy! Good communication equals good health.

20.

The Ultimate Truth Process

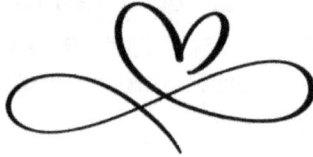

The following is a method of creating healing I have developed over years and years of study. It is so simple that now I wonder why it took me so long to get it. Perhaps it is because it has taken me a long time to unravel my addiction to Western medicine, and that had to go out first. Then I had to integrate all my years of Liberation Breathwork, my training in India, and what A Course in Miracles says. After that, I "reduced it" like a sauce.

There are three main parts to this self-healing technique. They are all based on taking 100% responsibility for our condition, and giving up all "victim consciousness" that blames an external "cause" for the condition.

1. Find the cause of the condition (the *real* cause, the metaphysical cause).
2. Confess the addiction (the addiction to those negative thoughts causing the condition) to God or someone.
3. Apply spiritual purification methods (to release the thoughts causing the condition).

The Ultimate Truth Process:

Finding the real cause of your illness is accomplished through *The Ultimate Truth Process* which you can do in writing. In this way, you become your own Sherlock Holmes, telling the absolute truth to yourself on paper. You must let go of the thought "I don't know," because that blocks your ability to access the information. You *do know* the cause of your condition. It is in your mind. You must just let the responses come up to consciousness. A writing process helps you do that. The following steps compose what I call *The Ultimate Truth Process* that I came up with. On paper, write the following:

1) The negative thoughts I have that are causing this condition are _____.

2) The situation that triggered this condition was _____. Or ask: The situation going on in my life right before I first got this condition was _____. (Perhaps you need to forgive some incident.)

3) My "payoff" for keeping this condition is_____. (A payoff is a neurotic benefit one is getting out of it all.)

4) If this condition could talk, what it would say is _____.

5) My fear of giving up this condition forever is _____.

6) The reason I do not want to give up this condition is _____.

7) I will let go of this condition permanently when _____. (What has to happen?)

8) The affirmation I need to think to heal this condition is _____.

Confession: Recognizing that the above data is an addiction (something I stubbornly hang onto), I confess to God and another person these above points. I admit that I indulge regularly in the above ego thoughts, and I have been refusing to let go of them. Read the points out loud to another person the above list you wrote, and standing before your altar, read it to the Holy Spirit. It is best to also read it to a Liberation Breathworker who can help you breathe out the *real cause* in a private Breathwork session.

Apply spiritual purification methods:

Affirmations	*Indian sweat lodges*
Prayer	*Fire Purification*
Reading ACIM	*Writing a Journal*
Breathwork	*Silence/Seclusion*
Chanting	*Acupuncture and Cranial*
Gratitude	*Sacral Work*
Meditation	*Visiting an Ashram*
Fasting	*Head Shaving*

Another process to do with your Breathworker or buddy is a verbal truth process such as a sentence completion technique. For example, say:

"I will allow myself to be healed when _____."

Keep repeating this phrase and fill in the blank. I am not talking about a particular time span. You are confessing what you think needs to happen before you are safe enough to allow yourself to be healed.

For example, "I will allow myself to be healed of _____ when I am sure my mother is okay first," or "I will allow myself to be healed of _____ when I feel I have suffered enough over my sister's death," or "I will allow myself to be healed of _____when I experience my perfection."

A skilled Liberation Breathworker would then take you deeper and have you say, "I will know my mother is okay when_____." Or, "I will feel I have suffered enough when_____." Or, "I will experience my perfection when _____."

These answers give the Breathworker necessary information about why you won't allow yourself to be healed now. Sometimes you may be setting up impossible situations for yourself, such as "I cannot let myself be healed because my mother is not healed." Perhaps your mother (or brother or other family member) does not want to be healed and you will have to wait forever! Waiting for family members to go first is a mistake. You go first and set the example. A Liberation Breathworker will help you process and breathe out unrealistic expectations.

The following is an example of the Ultimate Truth Process applied to skin cancer (writing):

Condition: Skin Cancer (Which I have had to process in myself):

1. The exact thoughts that caused this condition are:
   a. I am wrong because I could not heal my relationship with my sister before she died.
   b. I am therefore guilty.

2. My payoff for creating this condition is:
   a. I get to punish myself for that guilt.
   b. I get to prove *I am not perfect.* (My "personal lie.")

3. What triggered this the first time was: (My sister's death, for example.)

4. My fear of giving up this condition is:
   a. I would be perfect and that is not okay according to the church.
   b. I would be really happy, and I am not used to that.

5. If this condition could talk, it would say:
   a. I need to stay here until you get over your guilt.
   b. You do not need to keep me here.

6. The reason I do not want to give up this condition is:
   a. My loyalty to the family mind shows my love for my family.
   b. I am still trying to heal things with my sister (by copying her pain and death).

7. I will let go of this condition when:
   a. I will let go of this condition when I stop trying to heal it with my sister.
   b. I will let go of this condition when I am ready to give up the guilt.
   c. I will be ready to let go of this condition when I see my innocence NOW.

8. The affirmation I need to let go of this condition is:

"I am complete with my sister forever. We forgive each other. We are both innocent."

"Amen. It is done!"

I want to say a few more words to explain the meaning of *payoff*. A payoff is something that one gets out of a condition that is neurotic, or it could be something negative that one is trying to "prove" (the opposite). If the payoff is too great, the person may not want to give up the condition. To give up the condition, the person must also be willing to give up the payoffs. Therefore, it is important not only to understand what the payoffs are, but more important to learn that one does not need these neurotic payoffs. Below are examples of payoffs. Note that the word *symptom* is interchangeable with *disease*.

❖ *Attention*
❖ *Punishing oneself with the condition because of guilt*
❖ *Keeping people away*

- ❖ *Using the symptom to prove that one is helpless, bad, worthless, unable, not perfect, not good enough, a failure, and so on*
- ❖ *Punishing a mate or parent to try to make them feel he or she is not good enough or is bad, or even "guilty" for your condition*
- ❖ *Using the symptom as a way of holding oneself back because of fear of moving forward*
- ❖ *Using the symptom as a form of conflict because one is addicted to conflict*
- ❖ *Using the symptom as a way of trying to prove that there is no God*
- ❖ *Using the symptom as an excuse to be angry*
- ❖ *Using the symptom as an excuse not to work*
- ❖ *Using the symptom or disease as a cover-up or distraction to avoid what is really going on*
- ❖ *Using the symptom as a way of sabotaging one's life, career, or relationship*
- ❖ *Using the symptom as a way of deadening oneself because of fear of feeling and/or fear of life*

You can handle these issues in healthier, less neurotic ways. For example, you don't have to be sick to get attention, you can learn that self-punishment in the form of sickness is not necessary. You could forgive yourself instead. You could change jobs and find something you love to do rather than getting sick to get out of a job you hate, and so on. You can leave a relationship instead of getting sick to get out of it.

Following are examples of fears people might have about giving up the disease or symptom:

❖ *Fear that if one should give it up, one might have to be responsible*

❖ *Fear that if one should give it up, one might have to succeed*

❖ *Fear that if one should give it up, one might have to face something*

❖ *Fear that if one should give it up, one might have to move forward and be powerful*

❖ *Fear that if one should give it up, one could no longer get even*

❖ *Fear that if one should give it up, one would have no more excuses*

❖ *Fear that if one should give it up, one might have to be happy*

❖ *Fear that if one should give it up, one might enter a relationship and then have to handle love*

❖ *Fear that if one should give it up, one might end up alone*

You may think you do not have any fear of giving up the condition, but if you still have the condition, you still DO have a fear. When you work out the fear, you will be ready to give up the condition. The first step is to identify the fear and the next step is to give up the fear. Change the thought that causes the fear and breathe out the feeling of fear.

21.

Prayers for Healing

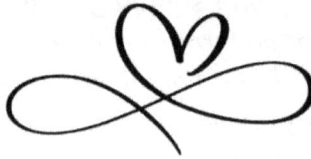

I am quite willing to share with you the prayers I use for healing, but I feel that you should ultimately work out your own prayers, so they have more personal meaning to you. It took me several years to get this right for myself. For me to get back into prayer, I had to work out my case with religion and all my disappointment around religious theology. After leaving the church, rebelling, and re-entering spirituality through Liberation Breathing, I had to find my way again.

When I met my guru Babaji, He allowed me to write to Him all my prayers in the form of letters. I decided that one purpose of a guru is to permit you to bare your soul to them. That is what I did. I shared all my problems, laid them at His feet, and asked for guidance. Usually, I had an emotional release during this process and my energy would shift. Then I would experience a change in my body. I did this for years; but now when I think of it, these prayers seem kind of crude and embarrassing to me. But it was the best I could do at the time, and it was my way of giving it to the Holy Spirit. Later, after Babaji entered his final

Samadhi (conscious departure), I continued to write Him letters, and still do to this day. I consider them my ultimate *prayer*. I place the prayers on my altar under the altar cloth until I feel the issue clears. It still works for me. But it works better now because I have learned to compose the prayers in a more responsible way.

1. *I state my gratitude to my guru.*
2. *I state my problem.*
3. *I try to confess how I created this problem myself; what ego thoughts, negative thoughts of mine were in operation.*
4. *I lay those at His feet and say that to Him.*
5. *I ask for the ability to see the problem differently, and I write down the new thoughts I have which are the opposite of the negative ones. These are in the form of affirmations (which are a form of prayers).*
6. *I ask Him to add energy to my new thoughts.*
7. *I give Him thanks for hearing these prayers.*

In this way, I take more responsibility for my case and show the Divine that I am willing to do something about it. I am not saying, "Oh, please do it for me." Begging for something is a lower form of prayer. Gratitude is the highest form of prayer.

Sometimes I add other steps. I sit before my altar and speak aloud to Babaji, Jesus, or the Divine Mother, and so on, all of whom represent the Holy Spirit's mind to me. At first, I felt silly doing this, but the results were fantastic, so I went ahead anyway. The desire to communicate with the Masters is essential to opening the door to their Presence. It must start with you. You must *invite* the Holy Spirit into your prayer process.

I learned a five-part prayer as a child in the Lutheran church that is excellent to this day.

1. *Opening*
2. *Forgiveness*
3. *Gratitude*
4. *Petition*
5. *Closing*

1. **Opening:** In this part, you get into the proper frame of mind. I do this by repeating mantras or by reading from A Course in Miracles text a few pages. You could also read from the Bible or from any spiritual metaphysical book that is important to you.

2. **Forgiveness:** In this step, you state the following:
    a. What you want to be forgiven for.
    b. Whom you want to be forgiven by.
    c. Whom you want to forgive, and so one.

3. **Gratitude:** Now you state everything for which you are grateful and everybody to whom you are grateful, with deep feeling, love, and appreciation.

4. **Petition:** At this point, you ask for guidance and help with specific problems. (Here I would read specific prayers for the healing of the body. See the example below.)

5. **Closing:** Finally, you again read some holy scriptures. Reading a lesson from ACIM workbook is ideal. Or you can read from another scripture.

Another way to do this prayer is to read the following at your altar:

> *Regarding my condition of gastritis* (for example):
> *I take responsibility for creating this with my negative thoughts, such as* _____. *I lay that at your feet. I allow you, the Holy Spirit, to undo all my wrong thinking that caused this condition and those thoughts that keep me from giving it up.* (Read the negative thoughts from your Ultimate Truth Process as a confession.)
> *I now choose to think that I can create peace instead of this. I place it all in your hands. I ask you to help release and raise it from me.*
> *I ask to be taught the right perception of my body.*
> *I pray for release from the fear of the miracle healing.*
> *I pray for help in the cause of that* fear, *which is my addiction to the thought of separation from God.*
> *I do not want to keep this error.*
> *I now ask (*the part of the body affected, in this case, intestines) *to cooperate and let go. I cooperate with you and follow You* [the mind of Jesus]. *I believe that You know what You do and will guide me. I choose union with You. I am willing to receive this solution.*
> *I have total willingness to have God's will for me, which is perfect happiness and perfect health. I know that in You, in Your mercy and will, that I will be saved from this.*
> *I therefore completely release the thought that this cannot be healed. The complete results*

of Jesus Christ now manifest for me in this situation. This is the time for divine completion!

If the above prayer does not produce results, try the following examples using your palms position as a symbolic indication of your willingness and desire to turn over your concerns to God.

Lord, I give you my anger at ... (palms down)
Lord, I would like to receive your divine love for ... (palms up)
Lord, I release my fear of never being healed of ... (palms down)
Lord, I receive now your certainty that I can be healed of ... (palms up)
Lord, I surrender my anxiety about my ... (palms down)
Lord, I receive now your peace about my ... (palms up)

When you do the palms-down and palms-up movements, spend some minutes in complete silence and wait until you feel something. Do not rush this process. Allow God to commune with your Spirit.

Note: Prayer *does* have the power to heal. Scientific studies prove it. Dr. Larry Dossey, co-chairman of the National Institutes of Health, has reported many studies in which patients have responded remarkably to prayer. In fact, prayer for patients resulted in patients being five times less likely to develop complications or need antibiotics. If you are very ill, not only should you try the prayers above, but why not get yourself on a prayer list and let people pray for you? It works.

I AM the perfect love of God.
Therefore, I am always perfect.
I am always innocent.
All guilt is gone. All fear is gone.
All anger is gone. All resistance is gone.
All unwillingness is gone. All rebellion is gone.
Therefore, I have no need for this condition now.
Now all symptoms are gone!

A Prayer for tough conditions or long-term illnesses

One has to study WHY one does NOT want to be healed. Try this simple writing process: "The reason I do NOT want to be healed is_____."
Then I suggest the following prayers:

Holy Spirit, I give you my stubborn refusal to let
you heal me.
I give you all my blocks that prevent you from
healing me.
I give you all my fear of being healed.
I give up to you my guilt that stops your
healing.
I give up to you my anger that stops my
healing.
I give up to you my fear of letting go.
I give up to you my fear of miracles.
I lay this all at your feet.

The following prayer is the most powerful one I came up with over the years. Recently I came up with other great ones which are in the chapter on healing trauma and PSTD.

173

Holy Spirit, I allow you to undo all the negative thoughts causing this condition. I no longer deny You Your ability to bestow Your blessing of healing onto me. I decree, I declare, I decide, I determine and I order, in the name of the I AM PRESENCE to let go of this condition. I know You can and will resolve this problem by offering me a miracle. I allow this. I allow healing to happen. I give up my addiction to fear, guilt anger and pain. I let go of my power trip of not letting anyone heal me so I could be king. I give up my competition with God. I give up the separation. I claim my true Identity is the CHRIST. Reveal the truth of this to me. I am forever grateful for Your help.

(Sickness and pain are due to competition with God. Wanting to be "king" is wanting to keep the ego and overcome God!) The prayer above is the one I used for my toughest condition (anorexia), and it worked. That prayer is really worth a fortune!

Further thoughts on Prayer

While in India at the dentist's office I saw a booklet on prayer. (Where besides India would one find that kind of book in a dentist's office?) I jotted down what the Swami Saraswati was saying:

Prayer is nearness to God
Prayer is turning to God
Prayer is fixing the mind on God
Prayer is meditation on God
Prayer is surrendering oneself to God
Prayer is glorification to God and Thanksgiving
Prayer is calling forth a spiritual force

BENEFITS:
Prayer elevates, transforms and inspires
Prayer gives peace
Prayer generates good spiritual current
Prayer produces tranquility of the mind
Prayer expands and purifies the heart
Prayer sharpens the brain and intellect
Prayer draws in the grace of God
Prayer opens you to bliss
Prayer shows you the next step
Prayer helps you attain success
Prayer changes your life
Prayer produces miraculous cures
Prayer works wonders!

This book, *Revolutionary Spiritual Healing*, contains a lot of my prayers. You need to choose the ones that work for you in your particular case. Prayer works, but you have to get the right prayer. After reading this book, and trying out the prayers you think are right for you, you should get results. If you don't get results, that means you need to adjust your prayers. Your subconscious thoughts are blocking them. We can help you find the exact right prayers. That would take a private Liberation Breathing session with us, because we would have to study the way your mind is "wired," and what are your thoughts blocking the prayers. Contact us here: bit.ly/LBSession. There is no need to keep on suffering.

22.

Breathwork and Healing

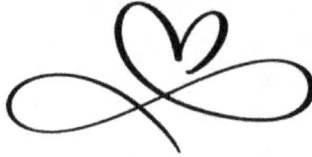

I was fortunate to be at the very beginning of Rebirthing in 1974 when Leonard Orr experimented with it. I was one of the first people he tried it on, and therefore one of the first ever Rebirthers in the world. I was only the 3rd person who had one of those first sessions at Campbell Hot Springs in California. Therefore, I am often referred to as "the Mother of Rebirthing," a title I wholeheartedly accept with the deepest gratitude for being there at the very beginning of this amazing healing modality. I was able to help Leonard perfect the process and spread it around the world. He and I wrote (I wrote most of it) the first ever book on Breathwork / Rebirthing: *Rebirthing in the New Age.* I had already written and published *I Deserve Love*, my first book, so I was well on my way as a writer.

In 2009 I was able to once again pioneer Breathwork, seeing to it that the work evolved spiritually into what it is today. After perfecting it and spreading it around the world for nearly 40 years, Markus and I were guided to call our form of Rebirthing: Liberation Breathing®. We added a more spiritual dimension to it. We added prayers to the Divine Mother at the end of the breathing cycle. We were told it's 9X more powerful.

Liberation Breathing, or conscious connected breathing, is a physical, mental, and spiritual experience. The physical part consists of connecting your deep inhale and exhale in a relaxed rhythm (with no holding at the top or bottom). The spiritual dimension of conscious breathing is the heart of the matter. One purpose of Liberation Breathing is not only the movement of air but also the movement of *energy* (*prana*). The dynamic energy flows that are experienced during Breathwork are the merging of spirit and matter. The energy flow fills your body with pure life-energy and clears your mind and body of tension and impurities. You can also remember and release past trauma, all the way back to your birth, with Liberation Breathing—which makes a huge difference in your life. It should always be conducted by a well-trained Liberation Breathworker. Only after one has become a Breathworker (or has had 10 private sessions and has passed certain levels of inner clearing) should one try to do this on oneself. The reason we do not recommend you try this on yourself right away is that something strong from your subconscious could come up (such as a memory from infancy) and that might be rather frightening. But with a Liberation Breathworker present, you would feel safe. They help you in the *letting go* process.

This kind of conscious connected breathing gives you a great self-healing power! We think of Liberation Breathing as the ultimate healing experience because your breath, together with the quality of your thoughts, can rapidly heal you. We have seen symptoms from migraine headaches, to ulcers, to sore ankles disappear completely as a result of Breathwork. Respiratory illnesses, stomach and back pains have disappeared. Frigidity, hemorrhoids, insomnia, diabetes, epilepsy, cancer, arthritis, and all kinds of other manifestations have been eliminated. Many of these conditions seem to have been caused or prolonged by birth trauma. Leonard Orr said, "People get stuck in birth trauma symptoms and then develop medical belief systems about them." He added, "Doctors can then become mother substitutes to support infancy patterns."

In Liberation Breathing, we see people go through physiological changes in ten minutes that other people stay stuck in for years and from which they may even die.

Liberation Breathing creates a safe environment in your mind and body in which symptoms from the past, such as childhood illnesses, traumas and patterns, can be released. It is a good idea to keep in mind that these symptoms are temporary and relatively easy to eliminate with uninhibited breathing. But if, in your mind, you are afraid of childhood symptoms or you resent them, you may inhibit your natural healing powers.

If you have a lot of fear, it is a good idea to consult physicians you really trust, as well as spiritual and mental healers, until you work out the fear of self-healing. They will help you get out of the traps in your mind. If you have a diagnosis from a psychiatrist, it is advisable that you consult that psychiatrist first to have their blessing.

Liberation Breathing is not for people who retreat from life in fear or who desire to curl up and die—unless they want to retreat from that pattern! Liberation Breathing is for people who desire to live fully, freely, and healthfully in spirit, mind, and body. We do not claim that any cure is permanent, because human beings have the power to re-create the symptoms. But permanent healing *is* the goal and *is* available. It is up to the individual to accept the opportunity.

Liberation Breathing's safe environment for mind and body enables clients to become free of negativity; however, processing negativity can be overwhelming at times. That is why we recommend you begin gently, starting out with only one or two sessions a week. We also recommend that you make the whole process of spiritual growth easier by STAYING with the process that assists you effectively and supports you in whatever changes you may go through. Cultivating the philosophy of physical immortality also gives you optimism and makes conquering difficulties an adventure instead of a string of bewildering challenges.

I could present numerous examples of healing by Liberation Breathing but that would require volumes to relate the complexities of all the personal case histories of people we have helped. But even if you labored through them, reading about them still might not help you. There is really no substitute for having a session and trusting your own intuition about your mind and body, and sticking with the process. I too often see people who had a few sessions long ago and did not stay on the path. Then they created some big illness and came back saying they wished they had stayed on the spiritual path with us. Liberation Breathing is a life-long spiritual path.

The purpose of the original Rebirthing was not for healing alone. We were trying to release birth trauma, but healing turned out to be a valuable by-product. When Markus and I started working together, we were guided by our spiritual masters to increase the power of Rebirthing by including a more spiritual dimension and to change the name to Liberation Breathing. Our sessions have five parts:

1. The interview and mental processing
2. The conscious connected breathing
3. Reading the Divine Mother names toward the end of the session while the client still breathes (oral breathing)
4. Closing with a powerful mantra to the Divine Mother (nasal breathing on side)
5. Working with new thoughts and statements that shift your mind to a new way of thinking.

The purpose of Liberation Breathwork is to acquaint people with a dimension of spiritual energy that they may not have yet experienced. When people experience this process, they can connect their illness or pain with the original negative thought out of which it was formed, and thereby take total responsibility for causing it. Some people are able to let go of the condition instantaneously during the session. It literally gets pumped out of the body with the breath. Others may gradually let go of it during the following weeks after the session. The breath is the cleanser of the body, as the yogis have always known.

It is usually possible to come out of Liberation Breathing in a perpetual state of health and bliss, but the path might be somewhat rocky at times. For example, when people re-experience their actual birth trauma in a session of Breathwork, they may also begin re-experiencing various stages of infancy and some feelings of helplessness. In my own sessions, I noticed that I never went through something I could not handle; the harder things came up only when I was strong enough to take them. But these rocky periods did not bother me because the more I worked out my birth trauma, the more energy I experienced. This kept increasing and still is. For the rocky parts, I was able to remember that "this too shall pass." Liberation Breathing ultimately raises your self-esteem, and when that happens, all areas of your life are affected positively.

I cannot fully explain how liberating it was for me to get in touch with the pre-verbal negative thoughts I had formed in the womb, during delivery, and post-partum. This is very deep work, and one has to be ready to face these thoughts and memories. A skilled Liberation Breathworker knows how to get a person down to remember these pre-verbal thoughts.

People may avoid this work because they experience fear when they think about working on themselves (especially thinking about releasing their birth trauma). The process does not add to your fear. One of the purposes of Liberation Breathing is to be LIBERATED from fear, guilt and anger. Feeling fear when you think of this work shows how much fear you have suppressed in your body since birth. Breathing it out will be a great relief. I personally would never commit my life to something that was dangerous! I have learned that it is more dangerous to keep the birth trauma suppressed. Even in a normal birth, there is a lot of trauma and negative thoughts formed.

The following information is taken from the book *Rebirthing in the New Age* that I wrote with Leonard Orr.

The birth trauma is your introduction to the world. It is the beginning of "The Universe is Against me" syndrome. There are preverbal thoughts and there is preverbal intelligence. Your thinking began before you were able to verbalize these thoughts – in other words before you were born. Therefore, when you were born, you were able to make sophisticated conclusions about that traumatic event. (Preverbal thoughts.) The womb is a comfortable place where all physiological needs are supplied. When we are pulled from this ideal environment, we experience a considerable amount of pain and discomfort. Probably a HUGE percent of our fear originated with the birth trauma. Some of the generalizations we might have made at birth are (preverbal thoughts):

❖ *"Being outside the womb is unpleasant."*
❖ *"I cannot trust people."*
❖ *"If this is what life is like, I don't want to be here."*
❖ *"People are out to get me."*
❖ *"I am damaged."*
❖ *"I can't get enough air (love), nourishment, etc."*
❖ *"I will never get over this."*

The birth trauma is one of the reasons most people don't like to get up in the morning. The bed simulates the womb experience. In the process of awakening, the memory of birth pains is stimulated to near consciousness. These near memories trigger the fear that you will have to re-experience being born again. Warm baths and showers also stimulate womb experiences. Some people choose even a hospital as a substitute for the womb or heaven. (Even something like smoking can symbolize being back in the womb, i.e., trying to get to the comfort of having the lungs full as they were in the womb.)

Impatience, hostility, and susceptibility to illness and accidents can sometimes be traced back to birth trauma. Many people feel either too hot or too cold and never experience lasting physical comfort during their entire lifetimes because of unpleasant birth experiences. We view the traditional theological description of heaven as a symbolic description of the womb. What people are really after when they seek heaven is to get back to that feeling of the womb. People want to go back to the womb because it has not been very pleasant since they came out; and it is unpleasant because of the negative decisions they made at birth, which produce negative results. The Breathwork experience was created to enable you to go back and dissolve all that.

However, not everyone had a pleasant womb experience. Some people have what we call "prenatal trauma." They may have had significant trauma if the mother smoked, drank, had a negative attitude, fought with her husband or experienced death in the family. In Liberation Breathing we study the person's conception trauma, prenatal trauma, birth trauma (delivery), and post-partum trauma. We call this information the "birth script."

We can figure out what pre-verbal thoughts you might have formed in each of these cases and how they affect you now.

Some people set up their relationship to be the womb. I could explain this convoluted condition, but instead I refer you to our book *Liberation Breathing,* which contains all the information you need.

The process of Liberation Breathing is available three ways:

1. Private sessions, which are the best, over Zoom or in person.
2. Group sessions, which we now call "Mantra Breathing," over Zoom or in person in seminars.
3. Water sessions with a snorkel, hot and cold water, obviously only in person.

We recommend people do at least 5-10 sessions for the full experience of the process. They can be booked here: bit.ly/LBSession. A single session over Zoom takes between 1.5 to 2 hrs. Sometimes less, depending what we have already covered and worked through.

23.

Other Alternatives

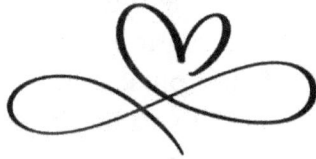

Emotional Release

I have found that when one needs to let go of any stubborn pattern or symptom, it sometimes helps if one can break down and cry at some point to get the physical release.

If one cannot get to a Liberation Breathing session to do this, there are other ways to get to cry and have an emotional release. One thing I used to do to make myself "crack" was throwing myself face-down on the floor in front of my altar and repenting my mistakes. Another way was lying down on my bed and talking aloud to Jesus until I finally let go.

Since I am a writer, the fastest thing for me is to write to my guru Babaji and confess my case on paper. You do not have to be a professional writer to write a confession to God. Usually when you get to the bottom line, you might start to cry. This cleansing helps.

Another thing you can do is sit across from a friend and say, "Something I feel sad about is _____." and "Another thing I feel sad about is

_____." If you are getting down to the bottom line and telling the truth, usually the sadness will finally manifest in tears, and you will feel better. You can often heal yourself of symptoms by having very deep crying sessions (especially symptoms of cold and sinuses). Feeling fear and sadness rather than stuffing them is one of the secrets of staying healthy.

To some people, it might seem easier just to go to the doctor and get some pills. But believe me, pills are only temporary relief. If you don't understand the consciousness factor that causes your symptoms, the symptoms can easily return, possibly worse than before. A Course in Miracles says that pills are forms of "spells" on yourself which do not work in the long run. Ultimately, you do not need pills if you surrender to the healing power of God. However, on certain occasions, if you have too much fear of spiritual healing, you should not judge yourself if you take a medical treatment. The goal should be to wean yourself eventually of that. Feeling and releasing your emotions is a vital key. Then as soon as you can, get yourself to a Liberation Breathworker! You can breathe out your sadness and whatever else is bothering you.

Movement

Sometimes it helps to say prayers and mantras with movement, especially if you can walk on the beach or on a relatively quiet path. It is very good to play a set of mantras (with earphones) and walk fast while repeating them. This really moves energy in your body and cracks your case. I find it much more interesting and effective than gymnastic workouts which I admit, I do not like!

If you feel too sick to walk fast or even chant, at least put the earphones on with mantras playing as loudly as you can and prostrate yourself in front of the altar, even if you must crawl to get there. That is a symbolic "movement" of humility. (See the section on "mantra breathing" at the end.)

I hope that you will seek out a Breathworker before you get too sick. By the way, if you have symptoms, don't cancel your alternative healing or Breathwork appointment. That is the exact time you need to go. *Get moving* toward your release. A good Liberation Breathworker can help you get through it.

Another form of movement that is not too overwhelming is to put on some music of African drums. Stand in place and shake your body, close your eyes and don't worry about how you look. Your breathing mechanism will be more open and productive because of that simple movement.

If exercise is too strenuous and inappropriate because you feel awful, maybe you should follow your intuition and not force yourself. Perhaps something as simple as the above will get you started. Later you can try something else such as sacred dance or an activity that has meaning to you.

I have also experimented with Watsu therapy, movement done in the water. I have found this to be *very* effective. I strongly recommend it as a healing technique. Watsu therapy is a healing art, and because of the water, the body can easily assume positions that would be very difficult to assume outside the water. The spinal fluid is stimulated in such a way that the natural healing powers of the body are enhanced. The therapy requires minimal effort because the Watsu therapist is in charge of moving your body. So, you could feel helpless and still get the benefit of the movements. After the session, you will most likely feel like moving again by yourself. It is a nice transition. Often when you feel sick, the last thing you want to do is move, even though it might help. In this case, the resistance is handled because the Watsu therapist knows how to move you, and the positions are not hard to assume under the water.

Jump, Don't Slump

We were in India recently with many of our spiritual colleagues and yogis. While attending the Navaratri at Babaji's Ashram at Chilianaula, near Ranikhet, one of our spiritual mentors gave us a good piece of advice anytime you feel a "slump" in your energy.

He told us that the calf muscles are a major center for generating energy throughout the body. When you build them up, they are as important as having a healthy and strong heart. Then he gave us a simple instruction:

Jump, don't slump.

Do a series of jumps in the morning as soon as you get up. This not only gets your circulation going, it builds your calf muscles and keeps your energy high. You don't have to jump very high. Just a little—a couple inches. We started doing this 108 times in the morning and we feel great the whole day! "Jump, don't slump." It was a great piece of advice.

24.

Diet, Health, and Healing

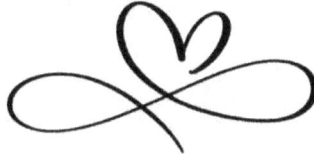

There is so much information available on this subject that you could easily read a hundred different books and get a hundred different opinions. You can feel crazy after a while, trying to figure it all out. For me, the subject of health and nutrition was one of the hardest things in my life that I had to work out for myself. That was because (*a*) I was born on the kitchen table, (*b*) I was born in the food belt of the world, and (*c*) my mother was a home economics teacher, so I had to learn innumerable "rules" about food that were supposed to make me healthy.

In the end, I rebelled against it all because I felt I was going mad. I had to write the book *The Only Diet There Is* to heal myself so I could relax enough to be able to eat decently at all. I was obsessed with this subject for many years. I tried too many different diets, too many ways of eating, too many food plans, too many nutrition programs, too many nutrition products. In the end, I could not think straight.

You must find out what works for you. I tried being a vegetarian. I tried being a vegan. I tried being a fruitarian. I tried eating whatever I wanted and not judging myself. (THAT was a relief!) I honestly feel the whole subject is best summed up by fellow immortalist, Joanna Cherry. She expresses my sincerest feelings better than I can. The following paragraph is from the chapter she wrote called "Divine Self" in the book *New Cells, New Bodies, New Life* by Virginia Essene and others. I recommend this book.

> *Are you eating what feels most right for you at this time? Foods are all thought forms, just like our body; and we do have the ability to transform any food – with our thought, love, light, intention – to a frequency that is totally beneficial to our body. But until we fully empower ourselves with this ability, our body will love some foods more than others. Raw and organic fruits and vegetables, soaked nuts and sprouted seeds and beans hold the greatest natural light. Many wonderful new substances are available today also that can enliven and lift your body. Try and just listen to your Spirit and the highest desire for your body and follow that.*

About vegetarianism, again, certain immortal teachers say that if you eat meat, you participate in the karma of killing, which does not correspond with your desire to be immortal. (However, it can be argued that is another thought you can change!) Other immortals say you should just eat what you want and not JUDGE anything! So, you see, you must just think for yourself. You must determine whether your thoughts are powerful enough to overcome these aspects, and you must decide how you feel morally, and so on. Becoming a vegetarian should be done from a place of love and as an expression of love. Then it is a good thing, but if it is done to make others wrong for not being vegetarian, it will imprison the mind.

You might need to consider this: if your thoughts are clear enough, you can drink poison and not die. But would you? Kahuna masters have done so. I met one who did, but most of us don't go around testing things like this. We don't go around proving we can drink poison. Well, then, are we ready and able to process poisonous food? Why make it hard for yourself? Which foods do you think are poisonous? Maybe everyone should read *Diet for a New America* by John Robbins. When you learn what goes on when meat and poultry are processed, you might not feel like eating it again. I suggest you investigate and decide this for yourself. Do not rely on what you were taught in school on this subject. How do you know that was the highest thought? It probably was not! Nor do I want to insist that my opinion is the only right one.

Here are some points of view from great minds:

Jesus*:* And the flesh of slain beasts in his body will become his own tomb. For I tell you truly, he who kills, kills himself; and who so eats flesh of slain beasts eats the body of death.

Buddha: Let the Bodhisattva who is disciplining himself to attain compassion refrain from eating flesh. Meat is food for ferocious feasts: improper to eat ... so said the Buddha. If, bereft of compassion and wisdom, you eat meat, you have turned your back on liberation.

Leonardo da Vinci*:* Truly, man is the king of beasts, for his brutality exceeds theirs. We live by the death of others. We are burial places. The time will come when men such as I will look upon the murder of animals as they now look upon the murder of men.

Henry Thoreau: I have no doubt that a part of the destiny of the human race, in its gradual development, is to leave off the eating of animals as surely as the savage tribes left off eating each other when they came into contact with the more civilized.

Leo Tolstoy: Vegetarianism serves as a criterion by which we know that the pursuit of moral perfection on the path of man is genuine and sincere. It is dreadful that man suppresses in himself, unnecessarily, the highest spiritual capacity ... that of sympathy and pity towards living creatures like himself ... and by violating his own feelings become cruel. And how deeply seated in the human heart is the injunction not to take life.

Annie Besant: People who eat meat are responsible for all the pain that grows out of meat eating, and which is necessitated by the use of sentient animals as food ... not only the horrors of the slaughterhouse, but all the preliminary horrors of railway or ship traffic, all the starvation and the thirst and prolonged misery of fear which these unhappy creatures have to pass through for the gratification of the appetite of men. All pain acts as a record against humanity and slackens and retards the whole of human growth.

Notice if what they said makes you angry. If you are still a meat eater, it might make you angry. These great minds would probably propose that your anger is a result of eating meat! Please do not invalidate my whole book just because you might be angry at these quotes. I did not say that you must give up meat. I am merely saying that it is a good idea to think it over and be clear on your decision. You might realize that you have been brainwashed by school, parents, television, and nutritionists. Maybe you have never considered your own spiritual feelings. Maybe you have never tried to be a vegetarian, and maybe you would like it. Who knows? I still like what Joanna Cherry said. Right now, we are in Estonia, and we were served elk which we ate without guilt. I am NOT being strict with myself about this subject right now.

I have been discussing food from a standpoint of health maintenance. It is also true that certain diets can help the healing process, but that is true only *if* a person truly wants to get better and is not sabotaging themself. My experience is that abstinence from food (fasting) has the most beneficial effect on producing healing. In my opinion, fasting is a very spiritual matter, and when done properly, a profound healing and a "spiritual gift" usually occurs at the end. You must process your mind when you fast; the mind is, after all, what makes you sick. Food is often used to suppress the very part of the mind at which you should be looking. When you are not eating, you cannot go on suppressing what you need to see because what you need to see will confront you. A good book on fasting is by Paavo Airola, *Are You Confused?* It explains all different types of fasts. You do not get hungry on the master cleanser fast, for example, and it works. Many other books on fasting are available at your local health food stores.

In general, eating less is very good for you. You have much more energy to help keep you healthy. It has already been proven that you live longer if you eat lightly. It is a good idea to start cutting down and to cut down more every year. But do it gradually. Some people, however, feel a real loss if you tell them not to eat so much. They feel a loss of love, probably because their mother showed them love by giving them food. It might also remind them of the sadness of being taken off the breast. For some people, food is like a friend, and they use it as a substitute for having real friends. The same is true for cigarettes. But once you get through these notions and get into the reality of eating lightly by choice, I think you will really like it.

Many people are just eating the same way their parents ate. They do not think of whether that is what they want to eat. Chances are that a new world will open up when you start thinking for yourself on this subject. Source your *own* rules.

P.S. By the way, if you want to give up smoking, I highly recommend the book *The Easy Way to Give Up Smoking* by Allan Carr.

25.

Clearing Karma

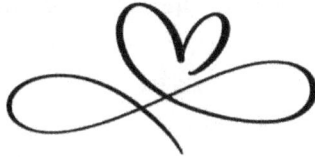

In the book *Star Signs* by Linda Goodman, there is an important true story. A friend of hers was shaken when he was told he had contracted a rare disease for which there was no cure. The disease, he was told, would gradually paralyze him over a year's time. What this amazing man did was to accept responsibility for his karma. He realized that in a former life, he must have caused someone, or several people, to be paralyzed. The action he took was an attempt to balance the scales under karmic law, which is quite impersonal. He thought he might have caused such a karmic debt by being a hit-and-run driver, running from the scene of an accident and leaving the victim paralyzed, or by deliberately injuring someone in a sport such as boxing or whatever. He thought that he might have been one of those in Rome who threw people to the lions.

Upon facing his karmic debt, he meditated on polarity action and made a decision. He resigned from his high-paying job and offered his service for a very modest salary to a crippled children's hospital in a nearby city. He read aloud to children, assisted them in physical therapy, and performed menial janitorial tasks. He began to forget about his own illness. Three months later, he noticed that his pain was substantially less. When he returned to his hometown for a routine check, the doctors were amazed to find that all signs of the fatal disease had disappeared. It was a *spontaneous remission*—the medical term for a miracle.

Another example might be that of a barren woman who lifts her karma. If a woman wants a child and is told that she cannot conceive or bear a child for whatever medical reason, there is often a karmic cause for her dilemma. She may have abused children in a former life. So, in this life she may adopt a child. Statistics as high as 75-85 percent show that women diagnosed as barren discover they are pregnant *after adopting*. When a woman learns the karmic lesson of atonement by taking in a motherless child to give it love, the karmic burden is lifted. (Goodman, Linda. *Star Signs,* "Déjà Vu" pp. 120-121)

Once I took a young man to India to see my gurus. This young man had serious intestinal problems and had a colostomy at a very young age. He consulted my gurus about this karma. My gurus were reluctant to tell him because they did not feel he would handle the facts well. He pushed them and pushed them to tell him. Finally, one said he had been a drug pusher in a past life and had been responsible for the destruction of the bodies of some of the people he had sold drugs. Later, he asked me what to do. I told him to work with teens to prevent them from using drugs. He did not like the assignment and got angry, just as my teacher had said he would. In his case, he was not ready to face the truth in himself.

Apparently, he needed more time to integrate this information. I was sad I could not help him.

Recently, one of my acquaintances from the "old days" of Breathwork was having an exceptionally difficult time recovering from her sister's death. She got sick and suffered terrible dizzy spells (which I did not know about because I had lost track of her). Where had she gone? To an ashram! I saw her afterward, and she was healed. She said it was the best thing she had ever done in her life. Initially, I was surprised she had gone alone, because she is wealthy and sophisticated; I did not think she would put up with spartan ashram life. Then I remembered that she had gone to India with me years before, so she had the power of ashrams built into her consciousness. She had taken our seminars and she had done Breathwork. Her Higher Self had remembered what was good for her. She did not complain to me once about the facilities. All she kept saying was that it was the best thing she had done for herself. She got healed!

26.

Seeking Spiritual Counseling

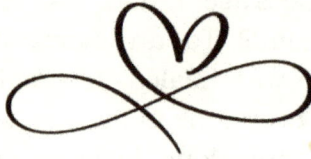

If you are stuck on something, it is often good to talk to someone who is more intuitive than you are at the time. You should always trust your own intuition, but when you are sick you may not because you feel "out of it," or you might feel that your intuition is almost shut down. That is temporary, of course, but when you are sick, your ego is roaring; when your ego is roaring is hardly the time for intuition. However, you must use your intuition enough to know to whom you need to talk. At least you need to know someone you fully trust who has experienced a specific healer, clairvoyant, or spiritual guide.

I became a great believer in trying many forms of healing because I didn't want to limit myself. I have had no guilt or qualms about consulting others when I have been stuck, especially when a past life was affecting me and I could not see it or process it by myself. Sometimes I easily figured out what to do or had a revealing dream. But often I grew impatient. Sometimes I just needed to hear what someone clearer than me at the moment could see.

Once I had intense cranial shifts that were not really headaches per se, but were painful. I knew they were important, but I had a difficult time. I was told by a spiritual guide that I was having exceptionally intricate work done on my electromagnetic fields, and as a leader, I must be willing to accept the ordeal. Had I not discussed this with a colleague, I may have gone into a panic. I might have felt I needed to run out and get an X-ray or something. By having this support and feed-back I relaxed, and I learned to know my body better. I learned to recognize the symptoms that indicate that kind of spiritual change and how they were different from other symptoms.

I must re-emphasize that you can get the answers yourself if you need to. In some situations, no spiritual guides are around. Once I got scared and started to think I was getting a brain tumor like my sister. I had terrible headaches and I became paranoid because such headaches were highly unusual for me. I prayed a lot. During the night, I dreamed that my skull was cut off by someone and set aside so that I could look into my brain. I knew I was seeing my own brain, and that was eerie, but I needed to see it. There was no tumor present, but there was a place covered with gauze. In my dream, I shouted, "What is that?" The answer came as this: "That is the negative thought you have had that 'something is wrong with you.' That negative thought is draining out." I was calm during the dream, but later I found it shocking that I had seen my own brain. Then I became grateful. I knew it was a gift.

Sometimes, a good psychic is needed. As I said, I have not hesitated to consult one if I felt that I was stuck in a past life I could not see.

27.

Benefits of an Ashram

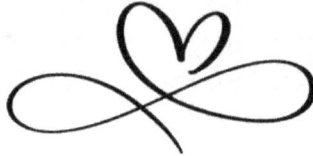

Since you are reading this book, I will assume you are committed to or at least interested in self-healing and are willing to do anything to stay out of hospitals. Let's hope you do not create anything with a serious condition; on the other hand, this can happen to the best of us, especially during highly stressful times.

If you want to speed up healing, especially if you think it is not working or is going too slowly, I suggest you go to an ashram. Naturally I would recommend Babaji's ashrams as He is the guru of the gurus. (You cannot get higher than someone who is able to materialize and de-materialize the body!) We go to Babaji's ashram every Spring to celebrate the Divine Mother Festival. You are welcome to come with us. It is a major life changing experience. I have seen people heal conditions there in a week that they had for years and years.

If you cannot stand the idea of going to the ashram in India, there is a great one in Crestone, Colorado. There are also several of Babaji's ashrams in Europe and other parts of the world.

An ashram is a place set aside specially for purification. It is usually in a location that is rather remote and "out in the elements" where you are receptive to more spiritual power. The central focus is a temple in which you pray, meditate, and chant for hours a day. The important thing about an ashram is this: not only do you have the energy available (thanks to the guru's grace, practices, and location), but you have a routine that is so different that it makes the ego collapse. Often this is just what you need to break up the pattern of sickness. Staying home, going through the same old routine day in and day out is often too "soft" on the ego. When you are forced to participate in a routine that is totally different in a setting that is totally different, you change; you are released, especially if the spiritual energy is strong enough. The rituals and ceremonies at an ashram help cleanse and purify your mind and body.

The subtle ego is hard to conquer, especially by your efforts only. A guru can transform your mind into a powerhouse of inexhaustible energy. You feel safe enough and strong enough to win the battle of your ego in an ashram. For example, I have seen people who were stuck with a lot of anger, which was destroying their bodies. But they were afraid to give up the anger because they had it wired up that they *needed* anger to survive. (They thought they would die if they gave up their anger.) This is not only irrational, the opposite is true, but the ego tricked them. In daily life, they were too scared to drop their anger. And yet, at an ashram they felt so safe that they became like lambs ... the sweetest things imaginable. There, for possibly the first time in their lives, they felt safe to give up anger.

I have seen people heal themselves of major life-threatening illnesses in an ashram. The constant spiritual energy pushed them through it. I have said the following repeatedly, and I still stick with this statement: If I had a serious illness, I would immediately go to an ashram and shave my head. I have done this even for illnesses that some people would not call serious, but they were conditions that were hard for me to heal. Rather than struggling and struggling with my ego, I shaved my head. This is brought everything to a "head" and cured me.

I had a student who had fibroids. The doctors recommended that she have surgery. She did not want to so I recommended that she shave her head. She did so, and lo and behold the fibroids dissolved by themselves!

Nobody is saying that you *must* shave your head at an ashram. Nobody is saying that you *must* *go* to an ashram either. These are merely choices that are available if you want results more quickly. The question is, "How long do you want to suffer?"

Usually, people have resistance about going to an ashram. They say they don't have time, or they couldn't not stand the conditions, and so on. That may be understandable, but what are your priorities? Do you want to end up in a hospital? Once you are in an ashram, it is actually very adventurous and fun.

I don't want to give the impression that you go to ashrams only if you are sick. Nothing is further from the truth. Ashrams are a place of worship. The more you go, the better. This is also the way to stay in bliss, to stay healthy. It is the best preventive medicine I know. People often ask where I get all my energy, and so on. Quite often when students go with me to India and experience the ashrams where I had my training, they later say, "I finally understand where you are coming from!"

Being around the great souls who live in those ashrams is exhilarating. They transmit spiritual energy to you all the time. Also, Babaji has trained certain yogis to do a healing technique called *jara*. You lie down and the yogi sits near you with a bundle of peacock feathers tied together. He strokes your body with those while repeating mantras taught to him by the guru. (The yogi can do this only if the guru says he is ready, and the yogi has prepared himself through a long and special process of purification.) This treatment is very effective. You can get this healing treatment at Babaji's ashram in Haidakhan. Why not come to the Divine Mother Festival there with us each Spring? Babaji told me once that you can make 12 years of spiritual progress in one day at that festival with those particular yogis, saints and gurus and with those particular ceremonies. Why not come and see that for yourself?

For more information: bit.ly/IQRay

28.

Quotes and Notes on Healing

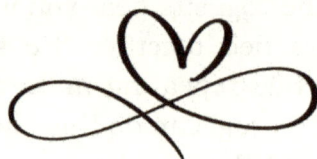

These are some of my favorite quotes from other healers:

Sickness always has an element of escapism in it.
Chopra, Deepak. *Unconditional Life., p. 9*

Complete healing depends on the ability to stop struggling.
Chopra, Deepak. *Unconditional Life., p. 24*

Spiritual connection is the hidden variable in health.
Ferguson, Marilyn. "The Paradigm of Proven Potentials" *New Sense Bulletin*

In almost all cases involving cancer, spiritual and psychic growth is being denied or the individual feels that he or she can no longer grow properly in personal, psychic terms. This situation then activates body mechanisms that result in the overgrowth of certain cells. The individual forces an artificial situation in which growth itself becomes physically disastrous. This is because a blockage has occurred. The individual

wants to grow in terms of personhood but is afraid of doing so. Often the person feels like a martyr (to his or her sex, for example) and is "unable to escape."
Robert, Jane, *The Nature of the Psyche: Its Human Expression.*, A Seth Book. P. 71

In cancer, a normal working cell decides that it no longer wants to function in contribution to the whole. Instead of being part of the support system, the cell goes off and builds its own kingdom. That's a malignancy.
Williamson, Marianne. *Return to Love.*

The following two passages are from the great book *New Cells, New Bodies, New Life* by Virginia Essene:

In brief, you are in a Holy Coordinate Point. Let me assume that these incoming energies bring healing to your soul and physical genetic body patterns. For this healing to happen, the cells must receive and retain more Light and be released of many past restrictions, limitations, and imperfections caused by the present life. The paired chromosomes must be cleansed at least four generations back. (pp. 2-3)

Health is an area in which everyone needs to claim responsibility for themselves. You DO have power over your body. From infancy you were told that you have no power over your body. You were told that you must always check with someone else about health and well-being. You have the innate ability to take charge of your body. You DO replicate your body daily. You create the same body because you expect to see the same body. If you wish to change it, simply intend that

when you wake up there is something new to greet you.
(p. 178)

I now give up death. I give up all aging of the body, all illness and any other effect that limited thought has had upon my physical form. I give up the idea of being any age. I am ageless and eternal. I give up funerals and funeral parlors and grave sites. I give up the idea of leaving life. I joyously accept eternal aliveness now. (p. 68; *New Cells, New Bodies, New Life* in the chapter titled "Divine Self" contributed by Joanna Cherry)

Illness is some form of inner searching. Health is Inner Peace.
A Course in Miracles, Text; p.15

The following are from Marianne Williamson's lectures and book, *Return to Love.*

Disease is loveless thinking materialized. Health is the result of the relinquishing of all attempts to use the body lovelessly. (A healthy perception of our bodies is one in which we surrender them to the Holy Spirit and ask that they be used as an instrument through which love is expressed in the world.)

Sickness is not a sign of God's judgement on us, but our judgement on ourselves. (If we think God created our sickness, how can we turn to Him for healing?)

Forgiveness is the ultimate preventive medicine, as well as the greatest healer. Illness is a sign of separation from God. Healing is a sign we have returned to God. By shifting our awareness from body identification to Spirit identification, this heals the body as well as the mind. There is a healing force within each of us, a kind of divine physician. This force is the intelligence that drives the immune system. The Atonement releases the mind to its full creative power.

The following is from "*No Law* of Healing" by Catherine Ponder in the book *Dynamic Laws of Healing:*

Denial is the first law of healing. Through denial you withdraw from your mind the negative beliefs and emotions that have played havoc with your health. If you can put a thing out of your mind, you can put it out of your body. Since denial dissolves, eliminates, erases, and frees. It is your "NO" power of healing.

Any prayer or statement that helps you say, "No. I do not accept this appearance as necessary or lasting in my life," is a denial. (In her opinion, to mentally affirm a healthy condition without first denying and destroying the negative emotions that caused your ill health is like attempting to build a new house on a site already occupied by an old building. Say no to an incurable diagnosis.)

Say, "I refuse to accept this diagnosis." (She suggests that you do not believe anything anyone tells you about your health unless they say you are going to get better!) Read chapter 2 of *Dynamic Laws of Healing* for further information.

In the book, Catherine talks about a friend of hers who was told that her daughter, who had speaking and hearing problems, was "intellectually disabled." When the child was four years old, her diagnosis was "developmentally delayed." Fortunately, the girl was not in the room when this diagnosis was given. The mother was told that the child should go to a special school. The mother told the daughter she was not going to acknowledge this. In fact, she did not tell the father, friends, or relatives. She sent the child to a normal school, and the girl did all right. At age eight, the child had to have an operation. The mother was told that the girl would never be able to have children. The mother again did not accept this and told no one. The girl grew up as a wonderful, normal person and had two healthy, normal children.

One must decide to stay in a beautiful state of mind!
(Tony Robbins)

29.

Pandemic Insights

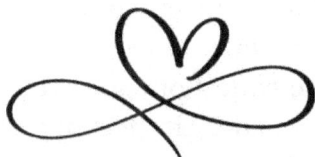

During the pandemic, I experienced some big changes like everyone. To stay clear, I did weekly Liberation Breathwork sessions on myself for several hours asking Babaji to be with me. Symptoms were coming up due to past lives. I did a lot of work on myself. In the process of Liberation Breathing, I received more information on healing that I want to share with you here. Some of it may be repetitive but it certainly won't hurt you to hear those things more than once.

The biggest killer of health is fear. Unexpressed and unresolved negative emotions cause harmful effects on the body. When one's self-worth collapses, one's immune system also collapses.

One should not go down to the vibration of the condition. There are many wonderful things to be done to stay high in vibration and out of the low vibration of the sickness.

Remain neutral about your symptom. Do not judge it or yourself, and do not get angry at it, yourself, or God. Love it instead and that will trigger healing. Say: "I now love this part of my body _____." (the area with the condition) "I am very grateful for this part of my body. It has served me so well." Example: "I love my digestive tract. I am so grateful for my digestion track. It has served me well. It can now be restored."

Once again, we will be healed when we are ready to be healed. One should say: "I am ready to let go of this condition. I have no more need for it." (Remember that it is wise to learn what *thought* you had that caused the condition, so you won't re-create it.) If one is not getting over it, perhaps the lesson has not yet been learned.

When experiencing a symptom in the body, one might tend to start a battle with it. There is another way. Say this to your symptom: "I am grateful to you for teaching me _____. I speak to you _____ (the part of the body affected) and I am telling you I got the lesson. Now you can return to your perfection."

One must give up anger at themselves to be healed. One must love their symptoms for the lessons they are teaching you.

All symptoms and diseases are an opportunity to process out the ego (which caused them in the first place), and for you to become more enlightened. Healing our problem or symptom is a way to get closer to God.

Christ healed people by not making the person's conditions real. He saw only their perfection. He saw them without symptoms. He saw their Real Self. Can you do that for yourself? The Real Self is in a state of grace forever.

We confuse our identity with our body and do not connect with our Higher (or Real) Self. The body is a communication device. It is a vehicle to get us to the inner peace we share.

The more we choose to feel good, the faster we heal. When we allow a continuing unhealed condition, it is hard to feel good, yet, if we do things that make us feel good it helps the condition to heal. We should train ourselves to feel good even when we are feeling bad within the condition.

Peace, joy, and relaxation are ingredients for healing. One needs to have certainty that they can totally relax and that it is okay to stay relaxed.

When we have a symptom in our body, it is the body's way of trying to rid us of something from our past. We must find out what thing from the past we are hanging on to, and then turn it over to the Holy Spirit.

Letting go of the past is easier than wrestling with the symptom. "The past is over. It can touch me not." (Lesson #289 in ACIM)

The condition is a "gift" to show us where we are stuck in our past and what we need to forgive.

All parts of the body are healed when we stay in the dimension of our perfection. Perfection is in the present, not the past. It is peace, not inner conflict. Perfection is God's healing voice keeping all things in our life safe. Say this: "I am the perfect love of God." You can also say, "Even though I am experiencing this symptom, I still completely love and accept myself."

We should say: "I now clear my mind of anything that would oppose my complete healing. I am ready for the Holy Spirit to heal me now. I allow it. I allow my body to reflect the healing of my mind. The Holy Spirit corrects all the errors of my mind with truth."

If one has pain, one should put one's hands on the area and say: "I allow Babaji to enter here. I allow

Jesus to enter here. I allow the Divine Mother to enter here. I put my perfection here."

Sometimes we speak the right words for healing, but the body must catch up. There may be a delay. One must forgive and not judge themselves if the healing is taking a long time. Judgement makes it harder to heal the condition. We must love ourselves and have gratitude for being alive instead.

` One must be clear that their desire to have their prayers answered is stronger than their addiction to suffering. The Love of God will heal us, but we must let it in. Doubt and lack of faith are tempting in a long-term illness. One must practice staying in certainty and faith all the time. Faith is healing. It seems hard to have faith when illness is roaring but that is when faith is needed most.

We must choose happiness over any payoff we think we are getting from the condition and affirm that we would rather feel God's joy in our body instead of pain and discomfort. Choose the joy of God. Let in God's perfect joy to replace the negative mental mass that caused the symptom.

We must be willing to give up our obsession with the ailment and be willing to come into harmony with the condition by being grateful for the lesson learned.

We never make up something in our body that we cannot unmake! ACIM says this, even about death:

> *Miracles enable you to heal the sick and raise the dead because you made sickness and death yourself, and can therefore abolish both.* You *are a miracle, capable of creating in the likeness of your Creator. Everything else is your own nightmare, and does not exist. Only*

*the creations of light are real. (ACIM; Text;
Chapter 1; Section I; ⁋24)*

During lengthy illnesses, one may think, "I will
never get over this." But that thought interrupts
healing and leaves no room for healing to happen.
Confess that to the Holy Spirit. Never say never. That
makes everything impossible!

Cancer is not really a disease of the body but
rather an inner disease. The real factors that *switch
on* cancer are an unhappy life, habitual negative
thoughts, repressed emotions, and hopelessness
within. Illness is a demand to grow spiritually.

Christ healed people by not making their
symptoms or conditions real. He ONLY saw their
perfection. He ONLY saw them without the condition,
He only saw their REAL self. The Real Self is not sick.
The Real Self is not even the body. The Real Self is
Spirit which is in a state of grace and perfection
forever. Try to remember not to make the symptom
real. If we give the symptom a label, (like a diagnosis)
that makes it more real, more solid.

Peace and joy and relaxation are ingredients for
healing. Of course, we also need the right affirmations
to correct the negative thoughts that caused the
condition. Affirmations are miraculous healing
thoughts. We must decide to think these thoughts
instead of the thoughts that caused the condition.

One needs to have CERTAINTY that one can be
totally healed. Faith is everything.

All parts of our body are healed when we stay
in the dimension of our perfection! This perfection is
right here in the present. It is in peace, not in inner
conflict. Perfection is in God's healing voice, keeping

all things in our life safe—and this includes the health of our mind and body.

We could say: "I now clear my mind of anything that would oppose my complete healing. I am ready for the Holy Spirit to heal me. I allow it. I allow my body to reflect this healing of my mind. The Holy Spirit corrects all errors in my mind with truth." One should even give over to the Holy Spirit the part of the body affected.

How does one get over doubt and lack of faith when one has a long-term illness? One has to realize that lack of faith and doubt where partly responsible for the condition. One has to learn to STAY in certainty and faith all the time and that will prevent illness. That is a state of consciousness one should strive to achieve.

We need to talk to our condition like one would talk to a friend. Interview it! Find out what pattern is behind it and be finished with that pattern.

One must make peace with the symptoms and not be in a *fight* with them. One should say: "I see the good in you. You are my teacher."

We may think a miracle healing is scary, but it is merely the body going back to normal. Feeling enthusiastic about something will promote healing. Ingredients for healing:

- ❖ Love of self and gratitude.
- ❖ Peace itself is very healing.
- ❖ Praising others will help heal them.

ACIM says: *"To give a problem over to the Holy Spirit to solve for you means that you want it solved. To keep it for yourself to solve without His Help, is to decide it should remain unsolved. The*

Holy Spirit's problem solving is the way the problem ends. (ACIM; Text; Chapter 25; Section IX; ¶7)

Markus on Staying Connected to our Source

During the pandemic we had plenty of opportunities to freak out. Sondra and I just got down to business and appreciated the time at home, and started to work more efficiently online.

We actually did better during the pandemic than we had in the couple of years leading up to it. It gave us more space to connect with our Source, be more focused on this connection, and reap the benefits of Babaji's *formula for happiness*: truth, simplicity, love and service. These four pillars were present for us more than ever during the pandemic.

We are not big TV watchers, or negative news mongers, so we did not indulge in the worst-case-scenarios that were circulating around. We were not so much into the "vax or non-vax" debate either, not speculating about conspiracy theories and behind the scenes analysis of what was "really going on!" We engaged in our spiritual practices as usual, that we would have done with a pandemic or not.

As far as what we did to protect our health, and prevent ourselves from contracting the Covid-19 virus, we took the advice of Babaji to recite ten rounds of "OM Namah Shivaya" per day on our mala beads. Ten rounds equals 1080 times. It would take us about 15 minutes to say them. We considered that a small investment of time to keep us safe, and it worked. Not once did we contract the Covid-19 in the height of the pandemic. We stayed clear. We felt good and healthy. And mostly due to our Spiritual Connection, we kept "charged up" with our Source Energy. We had a mild bout only later, after the first two years of the Sequester, when a friend finally came to our apartment and had it, unbeknownst to us. But it was a very mild case and it may just have been a "sympathetic reaction" to when she finally told us she had it. We were completely over it in only three days. We never tested positive for Covid, even during this mild bout. Babaji helped us to stay clear on this. We also read our Daily Lesson in A Course in Miracles, and produced a Podcast every day that we presented to a group of students who were studying A Course in Miracles with us. We published them here: bit.ly/PodcastACIM is the case-sensitive link.

Staying connected to our Source through some sort of Spiritual Practice in the midst of a crisis is the best thing we can do. This connection provides a protection, and builds our immune system. And if we are embracing this process properly, it feels great. It brings great inner peace and joy to us. Revolutionary Spiritual Healing depends on us nurturing this sacred Source connection.

Babaji said, "Work is worship; idleness is death." It is important to stay productive. This work, or "karma yoga," connects us with our Source more than anything else. And we love our work, so it is never a "chore." Worship is extremely pleasurable for us; so, our work becomes the same in this instruction from our Spiritual Masters.

30.

Health in the Future

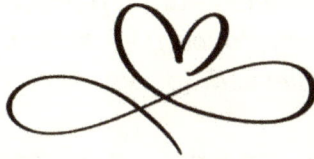

The famous futurist and predictor of trends, Faith Popcorn, says in her book *The Popcorn Report*, that self-healthcare is the future. We will become our own experts. We will counterpoint the advice of a homeopathist, a reflexologist, and so on.

Faith Popcorn predicts:

> *Medical knowledge and alternatives will cross cultures in a way we have never seen before. Homeopathy, Reflexology, Acupressure and Acupuncture, Biofeedback and Holistic Medicine will move from the fringes to the mainstream of medicine. Even newer-sounding approaches such as Aromatherapy, Herbology, and Ancient Indian Ayurvedic Medicine will be incorporated into traditional treatments or stand on their own as preferred courses of action.* (p. 67)

It is obvious to me that Liberation Breathing will be included in that list. She also feels that entertainment and travel will be health and longevity focused:

> Beyond health spas will be "Mood Spas," Universal Energy Gyms, Mind and Spirit Reunions, including therapeutic cruises that slowly take you to healthy places, in an effort to heal your body, touch your soul, and bring you back, twice blessed. (p. 68)

She says we may not yet be ready to admit aloud that our goal is truly to live forever—but we will pay anything to stay alive. (Well, I did admit it out loud!)

I wanted to live forever when I wrote the book *How to Be Chic, Fabulous, and Live Forever*. It was daring and ahead of its time. Many people never even found the book because bookstores put it in the "humor" section! When Markus and I got together we co-wrote: *Physical Immortality: How to Overcome Death*. We wanted to make the title totally clear.

Other reading we recommend on this subject is Louise Hay's book *Heal Your Body* that explains the common mental causes of conditions. And the most complete book we know about metaphysical causes of disease is *Messages from the Body* by Dr. Michael Lincoln. This is a must for all healers!

31.

Healing Trauma and Post Traumatic Stress Disorder (PTSD)

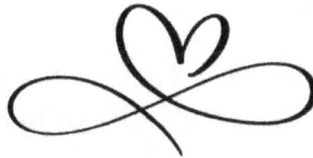

Be aware that this chapter could bring you Miracles! Even if you did not have a trauma, the prayers in this chapter will also help clear all conditions.

These are possible negative thoughts that can come up after a traumatic incident:

- ❖ I am damaged
- ❖ I am destroyed
- ❖ I will never get over this / I might never recover
- ❖ I don't know how to let this incident go
- ❖ I don't know how to let go of this fear
- ❖ I might not be okay
- ❖ Why did God allow this to happen?
- ❖ This is too hard
- ❖ What if my life is ruined?
- ❖ I am worried all the time now
- ❖ I have doubt that I can make it
- ❖ I cannot relax
- ❖ I am really angry about this
- ❖ I can't be happy now

- ❖ I cannot let go
- ❖ I can't let go of the thought I can't
- ❖ I feel really tense
- ❖ I am afraid something else bad might happen
- ❖ I don't know what to do
- ❖ It is impossible to get over this
- ❖ I can't be perfect now
- ❖ Even if I get better, this trauma might keep coming back

Although these prayers I specifically designed for healing trauma, they are also EXCELLENT for ANY condition.

Healing Prayers

You, Holy Spirit, have promised to deliver me from the hell I made. I hold you to this promise now.

I know You, Holy Spirit, are the perfect love of Christ and can erase all those thoughts (listed above). I allow You to do this.

I turn over all those negative thoughts to You, Holy Spirit, right now. I am giving You all negative thoughts that caused this situation and resulted from this situation.

I am even giving over any RESISTANCE to doing that 100%.

Every time one of those negative thoughts comes up, I remember to turn that one over to You, Holy Spirit, immediately.

If there is anything that would keep me from letting this whole thing go from me, I turn over THAT to You, Holy Spirit.

I turn over to You, Holy Spirit, any doubt or worry about all this.

I turn over to You, Holy Spirit, any fear that these prayers might not work.

I turn over to You, Holy Spirit, my obsessing about this.

I turn over to You, Holy Spirit, any lack of faith that I can be healed of this trauma.

I turn over to You, Holy Spirit, the thought that this will take a long time to heal and that this is too hard.

I turn over to You, Holy Spirit, the thought that a miracle healing of this would be "too good to be true."

I turn over to You, Holy Spirit, my fear of miracles and any fear of Joy.

I understand that whatever happens to me, I called for it. I attracted it with my thoughts (often subconscious). I was obviously out of alignment with my Higher Self.

I completely forgive myself for creating this drama. I recognize that I chose wrongly and I receive the lesson of correction.

I remember that the world is my classroom and other people are my "assignments."

I am giving up all anger, fear, and guilt around that situation. I let You, Holy Spirit, take that from me.

I am willing to give You, Holy Spirit, any part of me that still DOUBTS that I can be completely healed of this trauma.

I allow You, Holy Spirit, to restore my sanity.

I allow You, God/Holy Spirit/Jesus/Babaji/Divine Mother, to totally heal me, repair me, renew me, restore me, rejuvenate me, and relax me.

I can let go now, and I AM totally letting go now. I give up all judgement of myself for this incident. I am loving myself by letting it all go now.

I recognize that my happiness is a direct result of how quickly I can restore my fear back to love.

- ❖ *Spirit is in a state of grace forever [peace, relaxation, joy, healing].*
- ❖ *[My] Your reality is only spirit.*
- ❖ *Therefore, [I] you [am] are in a state of grace forever. (ACIM: Text; Chapter 1; Section III; ¶5)*

I am certain that from now on I am protected and safe and always okay. I declare that this will always be true so I can now relax and stay relaxed.

Fear no longer exists in my reality. The perfect love of Christ has cast out all my fears and continues to do so.

The perfect love of Christ dematerializes all my fear thoughts even before they can affect me.

Worry and doubt no longer exist in my reality either. I immediately let go of any thought that might cause me tension or pain in my body.

I EXPECT that the Divine is going to come through on my behalf because I have put this whole situation in the hands of Infinite Love and Wisdom and I have cast this burden on the Christ Within.

My Self-love is also helping me heal right now.

I allow the **Bliss of Babaji** to take over my mind, my body and my whole life now. It is happening. I actually experience that and feel that and enjoy that. I feel really good now.

I allow the **Joy of Jesus** to take over my mind, my body and my whole life now. It is happening. I actually experience that and feel that and enjoy that. I feel really good now.

I allow the **happiness and holiness of the Holy Spirit** to take over my mind, my body and my whole life now. It is happening. I actually experience that, feel that, and enjoy that. I feel really good now.

I allow the **Miracles of the Divine Mother** to happen to me now. I experience them. I receive the grace. I am blessed and I am very grateful. I ask for guidance always.

My sanity is now restored and I am getting happier and happier.

I am totally letting go. I am now free of all negative effects of that situation.

The past is over. It can touch me not. (Lesson #289 in A Course in Miracles)

Since I have in actuality given up all anger, fear and guilt, I am now able to be totally healed.

I am going to erase all negative effects of this incident from my body and replace them with my perfection.

I have ONLY good feelings in my body now.

This whole thing is OVER, GONE from my mind and body.

VICTORY IS HERE NOW. I commit to JOY!

I am thankful that the Universe is helping me to see this obstacle as an opportunity. I am grateful for what I have learned.

I know that when I align with the energy of love with thoughts, actions and beliefs, I am given infinite love and guidance.

I give You, God, all my gratitude in advance for this healing.

I now am even better and stronger than I was before that incident because I have cleared so much suppressed material in my mind.

Every hour now I am more and more relaxed and I feel better and better.

I am now aligned with God's Will.

Heaven consciousness is now restored to me (permanently), and I am aware of that.

I release to the Holy Spirit anything in me that would prevent these prayers from working.

When you begin to experience the change and the healing starts to happen, then it is good to start "acting as if" it is all complete. Then it is good to repeat those phrases as if it already happened. Imagine you are writing this letter to your best friend stating the following:

Example:

I finally declared this process completely finished.

After that, it no longer affected me, especially after I stopped obsessing about it.

What worked was giving all negative thoughts regarding it all to the Holy Spirit. I gave up all those negative thoughts that caused it and resulted from it.

I even gave to the Holy Spirit any secret resistance I might have had to doing that. I told the Holy Spirit if there was anything that was to keep me from letting it all go, I would even turn THAT over.

I gave up all fear that the prayers might not work to the Holy Spirit also. I also gave up all worry and doubt to the Holy Spirit. And finally, I gave up any lack of faith that I could be totally healed to the Holy Spirit.

I took responsibility for creating that drama and I forgave myself for creating all that. The most important thing was this: I remembered that Jesus said in A Course in Miracles that the Holy Spirit promises us that we could be delivered from the Hell we made with His help. That was very comforting to me. I held Him to that promise. The miracle began to manifest and I began to relax. My Self-love also helped heal me. Then I laid my whole ego at the feet of my guru Babaji. It did not at times seem possible, but I did finally manage to turn it all into a miracle because I also gave up my fear of miracles.

Then it became inevitable that it would all go away and it did. I went to the next level. I have remained in a state of supreme gratitude.

Final Completion

1) Keep doing the prayers until you get results. Print out the prayers that sing to you. Set aside an area in one room for prayer only and read those prayers daily. Read them out loud while

imaging Babaji/Jesus/ Divine Mother actually standing in front of you hearing them.

2) Cry if you need to cry.

3) Give up all anger about the event.

4) Do the forgiveness test on yourself. What level of forgiveness do you have on the people involved? What level of forgiveness do you have on yourself?

(10 is total complete forgiveness; 0 is none)

This next point is super important. What level of forgiveness do you have on the incident itself? (You may have forgiven the people but not the incident.) That is a subtle but important point. You must get to a 10 on all of these. You can say:

❖ I now completely forgive everyone involved and myself, with the help of the Holy Spirit.

❖ I now completely forgive the incident itself totally, with the help of the Holy Spirit.

❖ I now let go of this whole thing forever, with the help of the Holy Spirit.

❖ Forgiveness is the master erase. Give up all judgment of yourself. Judging yourself will keep the energy stuck.

5) You may need body work and/or acupuncture.

6) I highly recommend EFT (Emotional Freedom Technique) or "tapping." I have researched the best practitioners for you on line. Go to Linda A. Curran. When you see "images," click the one way on the left and follow her instructions. All tapping is helpful and free. But she seems the best for releasing trauma. Try the other practitioners offering demonstrations also, and find the one you like best. I especially like Brad Yates, who invented this healing technique.

5) Do MANTRA BREATHING as often as needed. (See in Chapter #35.)

6) If symptoms related to the incident creep back in the body try this: "It is easy now for me to let go of this trauma completely." Say this while doing the tapping exercises on yourself.

7) If you do not get results after doing what is in this book, it means you are sabotaging the healing. You would benefit from a private Liberation Breathing session with us to find out what your sabotage pattern is, and how to get over it. But you have to give up the thought, "Nothing works for me."

8) Always do a prayer of gratitude daily. "Thank you God/Holy Spirit for healing me."

9) When you experience some success, go out and celebrate!!

10) If you got over it all and then something unforeseen triggered a "flash back," or you re-create symptoms in your body, do not panic. Do this prayer instead.

I have given all thoughts causing this and all those that keep me from giving it up to the Holy Spirit. Therefore, it is easy for me to let go now. I give all doubt that I can be free of this to the Holy Spirit. I give up all resistance to being completely healed of this to the Holy Spirit. The Love of God and the Masters is replacing any tension or pain in my body. Therefore, I can now have 100% FAITH that this is complete.

I give up anything in me that would keep this prayer from working.

32.

Forgiveness & Ho'oponopono

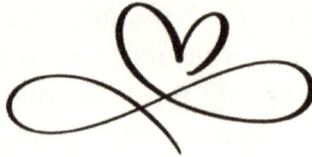

Revolutionary Spiritual Healing requires forgiveness. And this involves cleansing of the self we made up that has the "problems," which are spearheaded by "thoughts." These are thoughts of "separation" from our Divine Perfection. We need forgiveness to undo these thoughts and reconnect our awareness to our Source. There are two main systems of mastering forgiveness that Markus and I have practiced diligently over the years. One is A Course in Miracles, and the other is Ho'oponopono.

A Course in Miracles

A Course in Miracles was published in 1976. Before it came out, a friend of mine sent me the first chapter as a Xeroxed copy, with the hand written instruction in red marker at the top, "Sondra, read this immediately!" I felt the urgency of it. ACIM, as we call it now for short, is truly miraculous. It is a Course in forgiveness. It cleanses us of thoughts we are holding onto that are self-destructive, and puts us in touch with our glorious Divine Self. It awakens the

Christ Consciousness in our minds, and removes the blocks to the awareness of Love's presence that is at the Core Soul Level of our true Self-Identity.

The basic miracle of forgiveness is to replace our ego's (separated self's) thought system with our Holy Spirit's (Divine Self's) thought system. In order to do this, ACIM gives us a series of daily Lessons to undertake for a whole year. There are 365 Lessons in the Workbook. There is also a Text that supports the more practical Lessons with further clarification of forgiveness, and the awakening of our Christ Self within us. Forgiveness is at the root of this process of inner transformation:

> *Forgiveness is the key to happiness.*
> *Lesson #121*
>
> *Let me perceive forgiveness as it is.*
> *Lesson #134*
>
> *Fear binds the world. Forgiveness sets it free.*
> *Lesson #332*
>
> *Forgiveness ends the dream of conflict here.*
> *Lesson #333*
>
> *I let forgiveness rest upon all things, for thus forgiveness will be given me.*
> *Lesson #342*

Healing always involves some form of forgiveness, because all disease involves some form of non-forgiveness.

You may have a resistance to embracing forgiveness. You may think you are the "victim" of another person's attacks or an "unjust" situation that was not in your favor. Consider this from Lesson #134:

Let us review the meaning of "forgive," for it is apt to be distorted and to be perceived as something that entails an unfair sacrifice of righteous wrath, a gift unjustified and undeserved, and a complete denial of the truth. In such a view, forgiveness must be seen as mere eccentric folly, and this course appear to rest salvation on a whim.

This twisted view of what forgiveness means is easily corrected, when you can accept the fact that pardon is not asked for what is true. It must be limited to what is false. It is irrelevant to everything except illusions. Truth is God's creation, and to pardon that is meaningless. All truth belongs to Him, reflects His laws and radiates His Love. Does this need pardon? How can you forgive the sinless and eternally benign?

The major difficulty that you find in genuine forgiveness on your part is that you still believe you must forgive the truth, and not illusions. You conceive of pardon as a vain attempt to look past what is there; to overlook the truth, in an unfounded effort to deceive yourself by making an illusion true. This twisted viewpoint but reflects the hold that the idea of sin retains as yet upon your mind, as you regard yourself.

Forgiveness applies to seeing the false as the false. It involves the acceptance of your Self that cannot be threatened by external events. It asserts that your "original innocence" is the real truth about you, not the false theology of "original sin." It requires a Spiritual Identification that transcends a "body identification." We cannot be "hurt" at the Spiritual level. Therefore, it is important to get this definition of forgiveness:

> *Forgiveness recognizes what you thought your brother did to you has not occurred. It does not pardon sins and make them real. It sees there was no sin. (ACIM; Workbook; Preamble to Lessons 221-230)*

Forgiveness is a shift in dimensions. It sees through our Spiritual sight of a greater truth, and releases all illusory levels of false thoughts that are not existing at the higher, spiritual level. It understands that all pain and suffering come about in these lower levels, but it raises our awareness above them into the jurisdiction of Higher Thoughts. In this jurisdiction, pain and suffering do not exist. Forgiveness transmutes these "errors" of thought to the neutrality of zero valence so we can let them go. It corrects our "mistakes" by showing us our mistakes have no bearing on our Spiritual Reality, which is our only eternal truth.

In the World but Not of It

Most of us in the Western world, and even in the Eastern World now, have lives that are busy and engaged in actions that involve others. We earn money, pay our way, and strive to improve our situation, doing the very best we can at whatever we are doing in order to produce and maintain the greatest amount of happiness in our life. There is a part of us that we make up as we go along. And this "self we made up" has a complex of emotions ranging from sadness to gladness. Some of us have a greater connection to Joy than others. Some of us are affected by negative thoughts and emotions more than others. This is why we need contact with a Power that can undo these negative moods and thoughts that will raise our frequency to more positive vibrations. Our vibration is what attracts our experiences, and if it is low, it attracts stuff that keeps us more unhappy. Life wants us to be happy, and we have to practice the inner Life that will align our outer Life with that atmosphere of Pure Joy.

We have seen that fear, guilt and anger are the main emotions that keep our vibration low. They lead to despair, disease, and eventually to death. We have to forgive ourselves for sometimes falling into their pit of dysfunction. It appears sometimes we "cannot help it." We lose a job, someone leaves us, a project goes south, things do not work out the way we planned. There are many worldly situations that can throw us into the doldrums. But there is a Power in us that can clean all of this up and reset our course on the right track. We need to trust in this Power of forgiveness to set all things back in their frequency of joy and harmony.

The teachers of God [Love] have trust in the world, because they have learned it is not governed by the laws the world made up. It is governed by a power that is in them but

234

*not of them. It is this power that keeps all things
safe. It is through this power that the teachers
of God [Love] look on a forgiven world. (ACIM;
MT; #4; Section I; ¶1)*

How do we get in touch with that power inside of us?
It is the easiest thing when we are willing to admit
there is a frequency in us that we need to correct, and
we have the power inside of us to do so. This power is
what we would call "forgiveness."

1. Forgiveness is an admission, "I must have been
   wrong because I am not feeling joy."
2. I want to correct myself through real
   forgiveness.
3. I am not guilty for making a mistake, I
   completely love and accept myself anyway.
4. I am willing to see the thoughts I had that were
   in error and let them go.
5. I change these negative thoughts to ones that
   are more positive, and allow me to feel good
   again.
6. I invoke the Power of Love to help me do this,
   because I see the will of Love is for me to be
   happy.
7. I ask Love to add Its Power to my good thoughts
   and intentions.
8. Anyone who did things I did not like were just
   "acting out" my negative thoughts, so they did
   me a service in showing me what I needed to
   clean up and correct in myself.
9. I forgive all parties involved in this situation
   and see what I thought they "did to me" never
   occurred in my Higher Self. It is just a "Lesson"
   I am to learn by it.

10. I am determined to live in my Higher Self of Love and Joy. It is my ultimate Reality. My Higher Self is a State of Being beyond "problems."
11. I accept the Atonement for myself, which is total forgiveness of my ego self and everyone.
12. I am willing to give up all judgment—mine toward others and others toward me—and feel perfect happiness now.

This will for sure make a difference if you use these 12 steps. It immediately gets you out of "blame and victimhood" and puts you back in charge of your whole life. You can change your mind and change your results. You can reboot your mood and decide to be happy. You can take 100% responsibility and have total dominion over your inner and outer worlds. Then you will truly discover, "Forgiveness is the key to happiness."

Ho'oponopono

Markus and I have also been using the forgiveness process of Ho'oponopono for many years now, even for decades. Along with A Course in Miracles, it is the most effective method on the planet to master Forgiveness. Very much needed, it gives us the shift we all want—a restoration to Rightness all that is already created by Divine Rightness (but has temporarily gone out of balance), back to its Original Innocence, Perfection, and Balance.

This Hawaiian healing prayer process is a step-by-step approach to achieving peace, balance and a new meaning to life through the understanding of one's Self-Identity. It is a process to make right, to correct, and to rectify one's errors through repentance, forgiveness and transmutation. It is a simple, yet very profound, method of resolving problems and removing stress in a non-stressful way. It does not deal with the coping, controlling and management of stress. IT RELEASES STRESS.

It was discovered by the Kahunas (Spiritual Masters) in Hawaii. In the old system, it was required that the Kahuna (Hawaiian healer) was present in addition to all those involved in the problem that people wanted solved or healed. My Kahuna teacher, Morrnah Simeona, restructured the Ho'oponopono process so it works between man and the Divinity instead of man to man. It involves our interpersonal relationships, but takes the issues directly to our Source for transmutation and healing. In this way it bypasses all external interactions and utilizes that "inner Connection with Source" that provides the Power for healing and change.

It is a very thorough 12-step process. I cannot share the actual process with you here, because you must receive it from the lineage through which it came, which would be the "Foundation of 'I' Freedom of the Cosmos" that Morrnah left in charge to teach it. You can obtain the Ho'oponopono book only by doing the Basic I Class. Then you can practice the Ho'oponopono yourself, after taking the course.

Contact The Foundation of "I" at this address:

https://www.self-i-dentity-through-hooponopono.com/

The best explanation of the Ho'oponopono process was written by master teacher Ihaleakala Hew Len, Ph.D. who was Markus's teacher of the process. It is in the public domain, and you can download a copy of it from the Foundation of "I" website here:

https://bit.ly/HO-OPONO

33.

Fasting

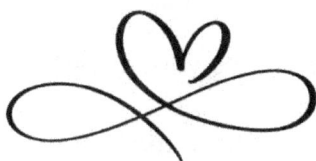

Would you do anything to get over your condition? If so, would you be willing to even try fasting? Faith, fasting, and prayer can produce miracles.

When a person fasts, his mental powers are heightened.

Fasting makes you humble and holy. It increases the power of prayer.

It increases your energy and reverses aging. So, it extends your life.

Since it gives you more direct communication with God...

- ❖ You will have more peace and serenity.
- ❖ You will have more creativity.
- ❖ You will get your questions answered.
- ❖ You will become more sensitive and able to connect with people better.

❖ Your intuition will improve greatly, with better clarity of vision.
❖ You will get more happy feelings.
❖ You will get a spiritual "release."
❖ You will get more spiritual power.
❖ Your ability to manifest what you want will increase.
❖ You can experience your mystery connection to the Holy Spirit.
❖ You will receive direction.
❖ You will feel in a wonderful state of worship.
❖ You will get the answers you are looking for.
❖ It will definitely accelerate your spiritual life.

Definitely consider fasting from TV and a lot of social media at the same time, so you won't miss the opportunities that come as *insights* while fasting.

After a death in the family we had a huge family drama that was terrible. It really, really affected me and I got some pain in my body as a result. I tried everything that usually works for me but the pain persisted. Finally, I wrote the deepest confession I could come up with to Jesus/Holy Spirit and Babaji and then I fasted on water six days.

The confession I wrote was this:

❖ I give over to you the thought nothing is working.
❖ I give over to you my addiction to guilt.
❖ I give over to you my discouragement.
❖ I give over to you all my doubt.
❖ I give over to you my karma with C.
❖ I give over to you my fear of miracles.
❖ I give over to you my fear of perfection.

❖ I give over to you my stubbornness and unwillingness to let go.

❖ I give over to you my fear of being totally healed.

❖ I give over to you my fear of being my REAL SELF.

❖ I give over to you all judgements of myself about this.

❖ I give over to you any fear I have of Joy and God.

❖ I give over to you my whole ego.

❖ I give over to you anything that prevents me from receiving your solution.

❖ I give over to you anything I have left out from this list.

❖ I pray for total enlightenment.

❖ I am doing the best I can and this is the deepest I can go now.

After writing that I "cracked" and broke down crying. That was the important thing. I don't think I could have gone this deep without the fasting.

The Essene Gospel of Peace

Aramaic scholar, Edmond Bordeaux Szekely, translated some of the Dead Sea Scrolls that were held in the Vatican. These translations were put together in a work *The Essene Gospel of Peace.* They are direct teachings from the *Christ.* The commentary of Jesus to a group of followers is very significant when He explains the benefits of the Elements and the practice of fasting.

The Living God Presence is something within us that can be known. In fact, it is essential that we make contact with it through a deep respect for the Elements. Jesus ascribes these Elements to the Divine Mother, which is consistent with what Babaji would say about them. Jesus goes as far in the Essene Gospels to call them The Divine Mother's Angels:

1. AIR
2. WATER
3. EARTH
4. FIRE
5. SPACE / LIGHT

Without a direct relationship with these, we are only theorizing about God, but not actually making contact with God's Essence within us in these dimensions. All Yoga insists that we honor these elements that make up the Physical Universe. When we do, we have dominion over not only over our spiritual destiny, but also over our place here in a physical existence.

The Earthly Divine Mother can heal us of any ailments when we develop this reverence and a holy Relationship with Her Elements, Her "Angels."

> *I tell you truly, you are one with the Earthly Mother; she is in you, and you in her. Of her were you born, in her do you live, and to her shall you return again. Keep, therefore, her laws, for none can live long, neither be happy, but he who honors his Earthly Mother and does her laws. For your breath is her breath; your blood her blood; your bone her bone; your flesh her flesh; your bowels her bowels; your eyes and your ears are her eyes and her ears.*

We first must acknowledge that the Divine Mother is in charge of our body. Her unconditional Love for us can heal anything when we are willing to turn to Her in humility, and request that all our errors in thoughts, words, deeds and actions be corrected. Essentially, we accept forgiveness for all of our past, and bring the healing into the present now.

Invoking the power of the Divine Mother to heal us with Her "Angels" of Air, Water, Earth, Fire, and Space/Light starts the process. Then Jesus strongly suggests for us to fast.

> *Renew yourselves and fast. For I tell you truly, that Death and his plagues may only be cast out by fasting and by prayer. Go by yourself and fast alone, and show your fasting to no man. The living God shall see it and great shall be your reward. And fast till Death and all his evils depart from you, and all the angels of our Earthly Mother come and serve you. For I tell you truly, except you fast, you shall never be freed from the power of Death and from all diseases that come from Death. Fast and pray fervently, seeking the power of the living God for your healing. While you fast, abstain from the Sons of Men and seek our Earthly Mother's angels, for he that seeks shall find.*

The most essential of the Divine Mother's Angels is Air. We could not live without the inhale and the exhale of this Living substance. To go without Air for more than a few minutes could cause our own death. Therefore, we must first invoke the Angel of Air, the Divine Mother's primary Angel of our Life Force and develop a relationship with Her.

Seek the fresh air of the forest and of the fields, and there in the midst of them shall you find the angel of air. Put off your shoes and your clothing and suffer the angel of air to embrace all your body. Then breathe long and deeply, that the angel of air may be brought within you. I tell you truly, the angel of air shall cast out of your body all uncleanliness which defiled it without and within....No man may come before the face of God, whom the angel of air lets not pass. Truly, all must be born again by air and by truth, for your body breathes the air of the Earthly Mother, and your spirit breathes the truth of the Heavenly Father.

We are glad to have Liberation Breathing because it is exactly what Jesus is asking us to do here. Also, spend some time unclothed amidst the elements if you can. This natural connection joins us with the Life Force beyond the mores and conventions of societal constraints.

Once we have invoked the Angel of Air and given Her adequate attention, Jesus mentions next the Angel of Water. This is very important. He lays out a water fast, and a series of colonic irrigations designed to cleanse the bowel and take away the impurities that we have accumulated in our gastro-intestinal system.

After the angel of air, seek the angel of water. Put off your shoes and your clothing and suffer the angel of water to embrace all your body. Cast yourselves wholly into her enfolding arms, and as often as you move the air with your breath, move with your body the water also. I tell you truly, the angel of water shall cast out of your body all uncleanliness which defiled it without and within. And all unclean and evil-smelling things shall flow out of you, even as the uncleanliness of garments washed in water flow away and are lost in the stream of the river.

I tell you truly, holy is the angel of water who cleanses all that is unclean and makes all evil-smelling things of a sweet odor. No man may come before the face of God whom the angel of water lets not pass. In the very truth, all must be born again of water and of truth, for your body bathes in the river of earthly life, and your spirit bathes in the river of life everlasting. For you receive your blood from our Earthly Mother and the truth from our Heavenly Father.

We are then guided to cleanse our bowels with colonics on a daily basis. You can purchase a home colonic cleansing board here:

https://www.therawdiet.com/colenzboard.html

Renew your baptizing with water on every day of your fast, till the day when you see that the water which flows out of you is as pure as the river's foam. Then betake your body to the coursing river, and there in the arms of the angel of water render thanks to the living God that he has freed you from your errors. And this holy baptizing by the angel of water is: Rebirth unto the new life. For your eyes shall henceforth see, and your ears shall hear. Make errors no more, therefore, after your baptism, that the angels of air and of water may eternally abide in you and serve you forever more.

Jesus makes one last mention here of immersing yourself in the Light of the Sun:

For I tell you truly, holy is the angel of sunlight who cleans out all uncleanliness and makes all evil-smelling things of a sweet odor. None may come before the face of God, whom the angel of sunlight lets not pass. Truly, all must be born again of sun and of truth, for your body basks in the sunlight of the Earthly Mother, and your spirit basks in the sunlight of the truth of the Heavenly Father.

In Summary, the three main Angels of the Fast are these:

The angels of air and of water and of sunlight are brethren. They were given to the Son of Man that they might serve him, and that he might go always from one to the other. Holy, likewise, is their embrace. They are indivisible children of the Earthly Mother, so do not you put asunder those whom earth and heaven have made one. Let these three brother angels enfold you every day and let them abide with you through all your fasting.

These elements are the "brethren" of the Mother's Angels, but also coming together in the Brotherhood of like-minded souls is more powerful a bond than even with blood siblings. He says about this:

It is by love, that the Heavenly Father and the Earthly Mother and the Son of Man become one. For the spirit of the Son of Man was created from the spirit of the Heaven Father, and his body from the body of the Earthly Mother. Become, therefore, perfect as the spirit of your Heavenly Father and the body of your Earthly Mother are perfect. And so, love your Heavenly Father, as he loves your spirit. And so, love your Earthly Mother, as she loves your body. And so, love your true brothers, as your Heavenly Father and your Earthly Mother love them. And then your Heavenly Father shall give you his holy spirit, and your Earthly Mother shall give you her holy body. And then shall the Sons of Men like true brothers give love one to another, the love which they received from their Heavenly Father and from their Earthly Mother; and they shall all become comforters one of another.

And then shall disappear from the earth all evil and all sorrow, and there shall be love and joy upon earth. And then shall the earth be like the heavens, and the kingdom of God shall come. And then shall come the Son of Man in all his glory, to inherit the kingdom of God. And then shall the Sons of Men divide their divine inheritance, the kingdom of God. For the Sons of Men live in the Heavenly Father and in the Earthly Mother, and the Heavenly Father and the Earthly Mother live in them. And then with the kingdom of God shall come the end of the times. For the Heavenly Father's love gives to all life everlasting in the kingdom of God. For love is eternal. Love is stronger than death.

Here you have the crux of the Essene Fast. You can take it for truth or not. I would not dismiss the power of a fast to heal you of ailments. Even the Medical Profession is looking into this manner of treatment now, at least extolling the benefits of intermittent fasting. Look into it.

34.

Mundan

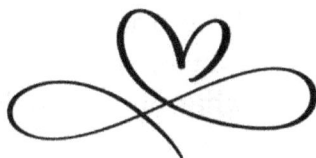

If you want extreme, rapid, surefire purification this could be it!

For conditions that are tough to heal, there is the spiritual practice called Mundan, or head shaving. (This includes down to the skin with a razor blade.) It is originally an initiation rite but it can certainly be used for healing tough conditions. It is best done at a spiritual site, not in a barber shop. The ultimate place to have it done is by the Ganges River in Herakhan, Babaji's ashram in India.

It stimulates all the psychic centers on the head and creates a singular unit of cosmic reception that has a clearer relationship with the universal vibratory state. This ritual has been done for thousands of years, so obviously it must be of great value.

Here are some of the benefits:

❖ It brings healing to the body.
❖ It opens up your crown chakra.
❖ It gives you deep inner peace.

- ❖ It processes your birth trauma.
- ❖ It processes past life karma.
- ❖ It helps you let go of old mental and physical patterns.
- ❖ It shifts your energy completely.
- ❖ It represents sacrifice of the superficial.
- ❖ It brings spiritual rebirth.
- ❖ It makes you a lot more creative.
- ❖ It gets you over what other people think. You have to rise above that.
- ❖ It opens up angelic channels.
- ❖ It connects you to the guru who then is responsible for your liberation.

Notice what comes up for you when you even just consider having it done. Imagine then how much you would process if you actually did it!

It is a very personal deep experience between you and God. It is something you choose. Nobody is going to make you do it. For me it has always been one of the most spiritual experiences of my life. It has always been a symbolic act whereby I am saying to God: "Look, I am going to try to surrender here as much as possible to You, and in this act, I am demonstrating that willingness."

At Babaji's ashram in India, the tradition is to leave your head shaved for nine months the first time (the period of the womb), whereby you are asking Babaji to take you all the way to liberation.

It is also recommended to be done if there is a death in the family to clear the unconscious death urge that gets activated. It can be done anytime you feel it is needed, such as for a medical condition that is hard to heal. Or after a divorce, etc.

I have had a Mundan myself 6 times in this life. The first time I did it was to surrender to Babaji. The second time I did it was after my mother died. The third time I did it was with Markus after we married. The fourth time we did it for one whole year together in order to accept our mission together. The fifth time we did it together when we received the spiritual assignment to move to Washington, D.C. The sixth time we did it together was after a death in the family, when we needed healing of body conditions.

I am not saying one has to do it that many times. For us, as spiritual leaders, we have an obligation to remain as clear as possible. Each time we have done it we have progressed tremendously.

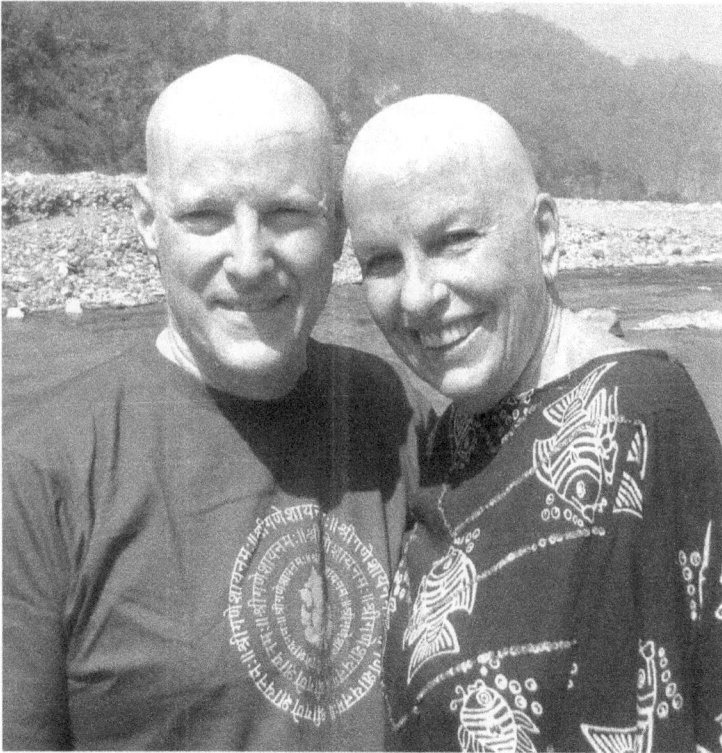

Markus & Sondra with Mundan on the banks of the Guatama Ganga in Herakhan, 2022

35.

Mantra Breathing®

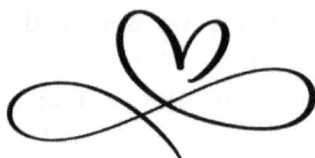

Besides the affirmations and prayers I have given you, I strongly recommend that you participate in Mantra Breathing with us to clear your body of any trauma or *any* unwanted pain or health condition. That is how I healed myself.

The mantra is a mystical formula that helps you enter a deep state.

- ❖ It energizes your intention.
- ❖ It accesses a high level of awareness.
- ❖ It helps to alter subconscious impulses, habits and afflictions.
- ❖ It gives you direct healing power of prana.
- ❖ It is a "mystical formula" which can entirely change a situation, your mind, your body or you as a person.
- ❖ It is a wonderful pleasing spiritual practice.

The mantras are for expressing our love to our Guru/God. The best thing you could ever do is sing praises to God or the Guru. Mantras are the highest thoughts.

Listening to, or singing the mantra will heal you. You can sing the mantra; but it is very, very beneficial to do Liberation Breathing while taking in the mantra. This is a double whammy. Babaji told me to call it "Mantra Breathing."

It does not matter if we understand a Sanskrit mantra or not. Listening to it, the meaning goes into us anyway. They are all praises to God.

The mantras can heal you. You can take the mantra into your hands and then move the hands over any affected area in the body where there is a symptom. Imagine the mantra going into the body while focusing on the Dream Team.

Taking in the mantra while doing Liberation Breathing will push out tension. Whenever you are feeling fear, that is a good time to do Mantra Breathing. It is more effective to do your Mantra Breathing with a group of people, because then the energy of the collective consciousness of the group helps you to heal, or break through an intention that you have.

It is especially good to listen to the mantras with headphones, and consistently notice how the joy of the music feels in your body.

The mantra will help take out the past if you are willing. Listening to the mantra while breathing keeps your mind in the present. In this way the past gets dissolved.

You can get good ideas while listening to the mantra. Have a writing pad nearby. I wrote a whole book while doing Mantra Breathing—*Outside the Box with Babaji* !

The mantra is God in action and is a very high frequency. Mantra Breathing immerses you in this frequency and you cannot help but to ascend. Mantra

Breathing is an ascension tool. You can get higher and higher when you breathe to these Divine Sounds and vibrations.

You can imagine the mantra going to the Divine Mother and She will receive them and send blessings down to help you relax. The minute you put the mantra where the discomfort is, the Divine Mother starts the blessing and the healing.

Mantra Breathing will energize your intention and help you access spiritually high states of consciousness.

Mantra Breathing will get you to your perfection. Mantra Breathing will lead your mind to what is important. Mantra breathing will make you more connected to Infinite Intelligence.

- ❖ Mantra Breathing will make you strong.
- ❖ Mantra Breathing will bring you to your love of God.
- ❖ Mantra Breathing will make you happier.
- ❖ Mantra Breathing will help you do a repair job on your body.
- ❖ Mantra Breathing will make you more alive!
- ❖ Mantra Breathing will make you more present and in your power.
- ❖ Mantra Breathing is very good for post-traumatic stress disorder (PTSD).

You should imagine that you are breathing in the energy of the Masters: Jesus, Babaji and the Divine Mother, for example. We call them the *Dream Team*.

Think this: "This mantra is making me feel good." (Which it will if you can let it in.) You can actually erase bad memories with the combination of

Liberation Breathing and the mantra. The mantra will become more and more comforting as you go along.

The more you hear the mantra, the more you will get cleared out. The mantra will clear you of anything unlike itself. Take the mantra like a drink of Divine Nectar—while unthinking whatever you do not want.

Think this: "The mantra is repairing my body, restoring it, regenerating it, rejuvenating it and making it relax." It is very pleasurable to hear the mantras. You will also get used to having more joy by doing Mantra Breathing.

Focus on the beauty of the mantra—let it roll over you like perfume.

- ❖ The mantra is stronger than your resistance. It will cut through your resistance.
- ❖ The mantra will obviously tap you into higher energy.
- ❖ The mantra will open you up. It will open your heart more.
- ❖ The mantra will stimulate higher thoughts.
- ❖ Taking in the mantra seriously is one way to let God take over your body.
- ❖ Mantra Breathing is like a lazy man's yoga.

It is also FUN to listen to the mantras or sing them. Doing LB with the mantra is like a fun sport. The challenge is to stay conscious on the mantra itself rather than have your mind wander.

The mantra will push up subconscious thoughts. This is good, but go back to focusing on the mantra. While breathing to the mantra, try to stay focused on the words—the sound of them in your head. If your mind wanders, say to yourself, "What I want to do right now is stay focused on the mantra," or, "I am staying with the mantra."

Pretend you are singing the mantra while doing the breathing. Sometimes moving the hands in the rhythm helps you to stay conscious, or rolling the body. One must prefer the mantra over one's mental chatter.

Why wouldn't you want to do this mantra breathing frequently as a spiritual practice? If you have an upsetting experience, do the mantra breathing as soon as possible after the experience.

After doing the mantra breathing for an hour, lie still in the silence and feel the clear energy in the room, and soak it in.

Here are the links to be able to access Mantra Breathing® with us. We have a two-hour Session of Mantra Breathing every Saturday at 1PM Eastern USA Time. We share & breathe to powerful Mantras.

https://bit.ly/MantraBreathing-1
or
https://bit.ly/MantraBreathing-2

I recommend you re-read this book again, and keep re-reading it until you digest it all. For further help read my book: *Outside the Box with Babaji*

P.S. Mother Teresa said that your only sadness should be that you did not become a saint.

36.

The Total Remedy: Atonement

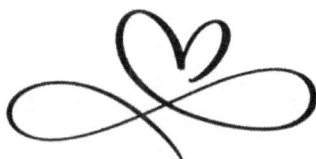

The Atonement is the correction of all our wrong thinking. It is complete forgiveness. It undoes the belief that we are separate from God. It is the decision to accept ourself as God Created us. The full awareness of the Atonement is the recognition that the separation never happened; therefore, there is no guilt or "sin."

A Course in Miracles has a lot to say about the Atonement. It leads us to forgiving ourself for everything, and forgiving everyone else for everything. Then our forgiveness is complete, which could be called the *Atonement*. The Atonement sets us free. It clears away all "thoughts that hurt."

In order to make this shift, it is necessary for some inner corrections to take place. When they have, we become more aware of our "True-Self." We become "teachers of God." Then we could say:

> *The sole responsibility of God's teacher is to accept the Atonement for himself. Atonement means correction, or the undoing of errors. When*

this has been accomplished, the teacher of God becomes a miracle worker by definition. His sins have been forgiven him, and he no longer condemns himself. How can he then condemn anyone? And who is there whom his forgiveness can fail to heal? (ACIM; Text; Chapter 2; Section 5; ¶5)

"Sin" is merely a term that organized religion made up to keep people stuck in the concept of "guilt." "Guilt" always demands punishment. The Atonement is seeing that there is no "sin," only errors in thinking, and all errors can be corrected. With errors, there is no guilt. There is no condemnation or punishment. This is a *revolutionary healing* concept that washes away the church dogma that teaches people they were "born a sinner," and that "original sin" is inescapable.

A lot of people today are not so conditioned or affiliated with a church. Religion is not so much in their life. But even though the church is not present, five lifetimes of religious conditioning can be carried into this one, and a pervading sense of guilt could be lingering even in an atheist.

Therefore, it is important for everyone to remember, **original innocence** is our only reality. All errors are correctable. There is nothing but innocence in the world of Pure Life, and only what Pure Life creates exists (in the absolute sense). Our egos (the sets of "thoughts" that imagined separation from our Source Energy) dreamt of guilt and condemnation. In reality even the thoughts, deeds and actions of our past that produced pain and suffering have no consequences to our True Self now. This Self remains pure. Our essence is pure. The Atonement gets us in touch with that Essential Purity.

This is the basis for these passages from A Course in Miracles on the Atonement.

Healing and Atonement are not related. They are identical. *There is no order of difficulty in miracles because there are no degrees of Atonement. Accept the Atonement and you are healed. Atonement is the word of God. Accept the Word and what remains to make sickness possible? (ACIM; MT; Section 22; ¶1)*

The Atonement, or the final miracle, is a remedy *and any type of healing is a result. (ACIM; Text; Chapter 2; Section IV; ¶1)*

Atonement heals with certainty *and cures all sickness. (ACIM; Workbook; Lesson #140; ¶4)*

All healing is essentially the release from fear. *(ACIM; Text; Chapter 2; Section IV; ¶1)*

When you are afraid you have placed yourself in a position where *you need the Atonement.* *The undoing of fear is the essential part of the Atonement. (ACIM; Text; Chapter 2; Section VI; ¶8)*

When you have accepted the Atonement for yourself, you will realize *there is no guilt in God's Son [which is you].* *(ACIM; Text; Chapter 13; Section I; ¶6)*

To follow the Holy Spirit's guidance is to *let yourself be absolved of guilt.* *It is the essence of the Atonement. (ACIM; MT; Section 29; ¶3)*

The means of the Atonement is forgiveness. *(ACIM; Clarification of Terms; Intro; ¶1)*

I [Jesus] am in charge of the process of Atonement. *"Heaven and earth shall pass away" means that they will not continue to exist as separate states. My word, which is the resurrection and the life, shall not pass away because life is eternal. (ACIM; Text; Chapter 1; Section III; ¶1-2)*

The Atonement can only be accepted within you by releasing Inner Light. *(ACIM; Text; Chapter 2; Section III; ¶1)*

I will accept Atonement for myself. *For here we come to a decision to accept ourselves as God created us. The Atonement remedies the idea that it is possible to doubt oneself. (ACIM; Workbook; Lesson #140; ¶1,6)*

The miracle is the means, the Atonement is the principle, *and healing is the result. The Atonement is the final miracle and remedy and any type of healing is the result. The Atonement undoes all error at all levels. (ACIM; Text; Chapter 2; Section IV; ¶1)*

The sole responsibility of the miracle worker is to accept the Atonement for himself. *This means you recognize that mind is* *the only creative level, and that its errors are healed by the Atonement. (ACIM; Text; Chapter 2; Section V; ¶5)*

Perfect love is the Atonement. *Worth is re-established by the Atonement. [When you are afraid. You have placed yourself in a position where you need the Atonement.] (ACIM; Text; Chapter 2; Section VI; ¶7-8)*

Your function in the Atonement. **When you accept a brother's guiltlessness you will see the Atonement in him.** *For by proclaiming it in him you make it yours, and you will see what you sought. (ACIM; Text; Chapter 14; Section IV; ¶1)*

Joining the Atonement is the way out of fear. *The Atonement is the guarantee of safety in union with the Sonship. (ACIM; Text; Chapter 5; Section IV; ¶1)*

Atonement is the end of Guilt. For you must learn that guilt is always totally insane, and has no reason. The Holy Spirit seeks not to dispel reality. If guilt were real, Atonement would not be. **The purpose of Atonement is to dispel illusions, not to establish them as real and then forgive them.** *(ACIM; Text; Chapter 13; Section X; ¶6)*

The undoing of fear is an essential part of the Atonement. *The miracle is an expression of an inner awareness of Christ to accept the*

Atonement. *(ACIM; Text; Chapter 1; Section 1; ¶26)*

Those who accept the Atonement are invulnerable. *(ACIM; Text; Chapter 14; Section III; ¶10)*

The Voice of the Holy Spirit is the Call to Atonement, *or the restoration of the integrity of the mind. When the Atonement is complete and the whole Sonship is healed there will be no Call to return. (ACIM; Text; Chapter 5; Section I; ¶5)*

The purpose of the Atonement is to save the past in purified form only. *If you accept the remedy for disordered thought, a remedy whose efficacy is beyond doubt, how can its symptoms remain? (ACIM; Text; Chapter 5; Section V; ¶7)*

Atonement is not welcomed by those who prefer pain and destruction. *It is extremely difficult to reach Atonement by fighting against sin. (ACIM; Text; Chapter 18; Section VII; ¶1)*

The Atonement is the one need in this world that is universal. *The full awareness of the Atonement is the recognition that the separation never occurred. [If you get THAT, you are not guilty.] (ACIM; Text; Chapter 6; Section II; ¶5)*

You cannot abide in peace unless you accept the Atonement for yourself, *because the Atonement is the way to peace. (ACIM; Text; Chapter 9; Section VII; ¶2)*

When you have accepted the Atonement for yourself, you will realize that there is no guilt in God's Son. **Accepting the Atonement for yourself teaches you what Immortality is.** *(ACIM; Text; Chapter 13; Section I; ¶9)*

The Atonement is the final lesson he need learn, *for it teaches him that, never having sinned, he has no need of salvation. (ACIM; Text; Chapter 13; Intro; ¶4)*

Atonement heals with certainty and cures all sickness and pain. *(ACIM, Workbook; Lesson #140; ¶4)*

Atonement means correction and undoing of all errors. *When this has been accomplished, the teacher of God becomes a miracle worker. His sins have been forgiven him. (ACIM; Manual for Teachers; Section 18; ¶4)*

All fear is ultimately reducible to the basic misperception that you have the ability to usurp the power of God. Of course, you neither can nor have been able to do this. **Here is the real basis for your escape from fear. The escape is brought about by your acceptance of the Atonement,** *which enables you to realize that your errors never really occurred. (ACIM; Text; Chapter 2; Section I; ¶4)*

The Atonement does not make Holy. You were created Holy. *It merely brings unholiness to holiness. The Atonement is so gentle, you* *need but whisper and all its power will rush to your assistance and support. The Atonement offers you God! (ACIM; Text; Chapter 14; Section IX; ¶1,3)*

But the Atonement restores Spirit to its proper place. *The mind that serves Spirit is invulnerable. The purpose of the Atonement is to restore everything to you. (ACIM; Text; Chapter 1; Section IV; ¶2)*

Excluding yourself from the Atonement is the ego's last-ditch defense of its own existence. *Give this error over to the Holy Spirit. (ACIM; Text; Chapter 5; Section VII; ¶3)*

Atonement might be equated with total escape from the past and total lack of interest in the future. Heaven is here. There is nowhere else. Heaven is now. There is no other time*. No teaching that does not lead to this is of concern to God's teachers. (ACIM; Manual for Teachers; Section 24; ¶6)*

Accepting the Atonement for yourself means not to give support to someone's dream of sickness and of death. *It means that you share not his wish to separate, and let him turn illusions on himself. Nor do you wish that they be turned, instead, on you. (ACIM; Text; Chapter 28; Section IV; ¶1)*

Every minute and every second gives you a chance to save yourself*.... Yet you cannot abide in peace unless you accept the Atonement,* *because the Atonement is the way to peace. (ACIM; Text; Chapter 9; Section VII; ¶1, 2)*

*If the sole responsibility of the miracle worker is to accept the Atonement for himself, and I assure you that it is, then the responsibility for what is atoned for cannot be yours. **The dilemma cannot be resolved except by accepting the solution of undoing.** (ACIM; Text; Chapter 5; Section V; ¶7)*

The Atonement is enlightenment.

The Atonement makes you sharper and sharper.

The more you accept the Atonement for yourself, the happier you will be.

The Atonement is a gift you give to yourself.

The Atonement is choosing bliss for yourself.

You can now *experience the realization* of the Atonement. You can now experience the love and joy the Atonement brings.

Forgiveness, Salvation and Atonement are all one.
Ask the Holy Spirit to help you accept the Atonement for yourself.

Comment:

Consequently, the miracle joins us with the Atonement by placing the mind in the service of the Holy Spirit. The Atonement is WAKING UP and realizing that "sin" could not happen, and never happened. My teacher, Ken Wapnick, called the Atonement the Holy Spirit's plan to undo the ego and heal the belief in separation. It is also the realization that we can and will forgive ourselves and our brother completely.

Repeat this very often:

I will accept Atonement for myself. *Lesson #139*

In summary:

- ❖ The Atonement is the correction of all your wrong thinking.
- ❖ The Atonement is total forgiveness of yourself.
- ❖ The Atonement is the end of guilt forever.
- ❖ The Atonement is perfect love.
- ❖ The Atonement is how your worth is re-instated.
- ❖ The Atonement is the way to Peace.
- ❖ The Atonement is the return to your Real Self.
- ❖ The Atonement is the key to happiness.
- ❖ The Atonement is complete forgiveness of all "others."
- ❖ Atonement is *Revolutionary Spiritual Healing.*
- ❖ The Atonement is the doorway to "Heaven on Earth."

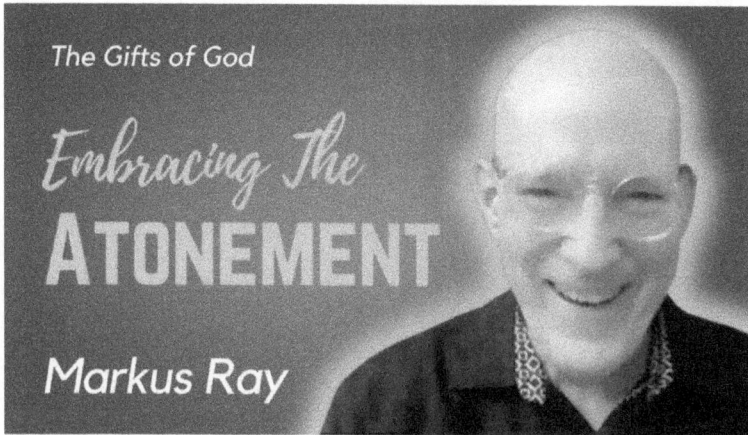

The Gifts of God

Embracing The
ATONEMENT

Markus Ray

A "Gifts of God Program" lecture on YouTube:

https://youtu.be/w81SQsohk7U

37.

My Summary of Healing

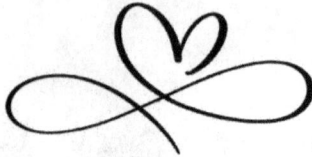

You will be healed when you are ready to be healed. You will be ready to be healed when you believe you deserve it. You will believe you deserve it when you are ready to stop punishing yourself. You will stop punishing yourself when you give up guilt. You will give up guilt when you believe you are innocent. You will see you are innocent when you remember who you are. You will remember who you are when you stop making up the ego. You will stop making up the ego when you want bliss and peace more than anything else. You will want bliss and peace when you are sick of being sick and when you see what a waste of time it is to be in hell. The choice is yours. (One teacher said you must want liberation as much as a drowning person wants air.)

Permanent healing means going back to who and what you really are. It is easy and natural; the only reason it *seems* hard is because you must let go of addictions—addictions to thoughts that cause conditions of illness. It seems hard to give up addictions because you think they control you and that you are not in control of them. In my opinion, an addiction to a way of thinking is a stubborn refusal to give up a thought causing your condition. When you face your stubbornness and refusal as being something you choose, you know you can choose otherwise.

A Course in Miracles says that you must say, "I see no more value in this." That means you must also admit that you get payoff from your pain or illness. You receive a kind of neurotic value out of this condition, and now you must be willing to give up that payoff. For example, maybe you must decide you don't need this symptom anymore to get attention. You no longer need this symptom to punish yourself. You have enjoyed enough attention and you feel punished enough! Perhaps you have learned you can get attention in a healthier way. or perhaps you feel you have balanced your karma and you can go on to something else.

But what if you could forgive yourself *sooner?* Then you would not have to punish yourself for so long. To forgive yourself sooner requires a basic understanding of who you are: You are *love* and your sins are not real. You must know that you are not a bad person. You are actually magnificent. You are a child of God. You are divine. You are not a sinner. Your disasters are not sins; they are mistakes. A mistake means "missing the mark." A mistake is a slip when you temporarily forget who you are. God does not make your errors real, because God knows you were just having a nightmare. Nightmares are not real. The ego is a nightmare. But since the ego is not real, the error is not real. Therefore, you do not deserve to be punished and you do not need to create illnesses as a form of punishment. If God does not make your mistakes real, why should you? You are innocent. Affirm that innocence is the answer.

- ❖ *Since I am innocent, I do not need to suffer.*
- ❖ *Since I am innocent, I deserve to be healed.*
- ❖ *Since I am innocent, I can let go of all the pain and disease in my mind and body.*
- ❖ *Since I am innocent, the Holy Spirit in me knows the solution.*
- ❖ *Since I am innocent, it is safe, right, and holy to have a perfectly functioning body.*
- ❖ *Since I am innocent, I can be happy.*
- ❖ *Since I am innocent, I can give myself love and keep it.*
- ❖ *Since I am innocent, I can have all that I need and want.*
- ❖ *Since I am innocent, I can handle a lot of energy.*
- ❖ *Since I am innocent, I can trust myself to do the right thing.*
- ❖ *Since I am innocent, I can be defenseless.*
- ❖ *Since I am innocent, I am at peace.*
- ❖ *Since I am innocent, my body responds to feeling good.*
- ❖ *Since I am innocent, I can totally relax.*
- ❖ *Since I am innocent, I can become wiser.*
- ❖ *Since I am innocent, I can say "no" without losing people's love.*
- ❖ *Since I am innocent, I can enjoy food, money, and sex.*
- ❖ *Since I am innocent, I can enjoy everything.*
- ❖ *Since I am innocent, it is okay to have material things that make me feel good.*
- ❖ *Since I am innocent, I have nothing to worry about.*

- ❖ *Since I am innocent, I can leave situations that are not good for me.*
- ❖ *Since I am innocent, fun is natural.*
- ❖ *Since I am innocent, life is natural.*
- ❖ *Since I am innocent, success is natural.*
- ❖ *Since I am innocent, I do not have to age and die and punish myself.*
- ❖ *Since I am innocent, I can live as long as I choose while improving my body.*
- ❖ *Since I am innocent, I can be in the kingdom of heaven here and now.*
- ❖ *Since I am innocent, I can be close to spiritual masters.*
- ❖ *Since I am innocent, I can make big contributions to humanity.*

Blessings of healing to you. Love, Sondra Ray!

An Invitation

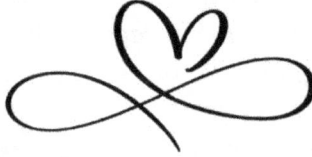

If you would like Markus Ray and me to speak in your community, your workplace, or at any public event or conference, visit us at www.SondraRay.com. If you are interested in traveling with us on spiritual trips we call "Quests," please contact us at the website address.

- ❖ In December - Travel to Bali with us to visit sacred sites and to enhance your physical immortality. (**bit.ly/BQRay**)
- ❖ In the Spring (March/April) - Travel to India with us and deepen your connection to the Divine Mother. (**bit.ly/IQRay**)
- ❖ Other quests to be announced (**bit.ly/EventsRay**)

Markus and I look forward to meeting you in person.

Thank You

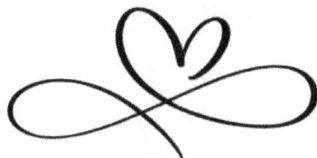

Thank you for telling others about this book. A Course in Miracles says, "Nothing real can be increased except by sharing."

If you tell someone who is ill or suffering about this book, they will be very grateful to you. Even if you tell someone about it who is not ill, they will learn how to prevent illnesses, so they will be grateful to you as well. This book also makes an excellent GIFT.

Love,

Sondra Ray

An Intro To "My Most Difficult Initiations As a Healer"

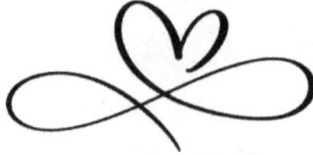

Much constructive debate between Barbara, our editor, Sondra, and myself took place to consider the inclusion or exclusion of this final section: "My Most Difficult Initiations as a Healer." Even the fact it is "set apart" from the rest of the body of *Revolutionary Spiritual Healing* was keenly considered.

In it, Sondra presents some of the physical and metaphysical "trials" she went through in her conviction to be fully with her mission in this life as a spiritual leader, teacher, and healer. It presents the "teacher" in her most shaky moments as a "student" herself of this inner work. Vulnerable indeed it is.

A certain amount of vulnerability is necessary for *Revolutionary Spiritual Healing* to work. Faith is tested. Already, *RSH* is a direction not "main stream" in the practices of most in the medical / big Pharma industrial complex. By including this story, we are "sticking our neck out," as Sondra Ray has often done, embracing this vulnerability and including it in our own evolutionary (and Atonement) process. We want to give you, our readers, a clear view that vulnerability is a good thing, an honest assessment of the challenges we all go through to grow and evolve in our Ascension to be our True Self.

Is some of it "phantasmagorical?" Indeed, yes again. Is there a fine line between "truth" and "fantasy?" I suppose again, yes. Did Sondra actually go through these things? I have never known her to just "make stuff up" for effect. So, "yes" to that one too.

Does it present her in what could be deemed a "crazy light?" Such spiritual giants as Babaji, who manifested his body out of light in a remote Himalayan cave, or Dr. Schucman, a Ph.D. professor at Columbia University channeling messages from Jesus in a back room of her usually prestigious academic bastion of "knowledge-based," tenure-tracked professionals, would be otherwise dismissed as well—in that "crazy light." We ask you, kind reader, to forgo any premature judgments of the far-fetched. Including this section, we err on the side of good spiritual company, who could also be deemed dangerously close to that *lunatic fringe.*

The *RSH* message is simple, though, not in error at all: the mind, more powerful than we are all willing to admit I suppose, is the *prerequisite cause* of all illness and subsequent cure. If it is "revolutionary" to see this fact, and posit it as simply put in *RSH*, then so be it. Forgiveness would then become a necessity for us not to pass judgment over the mistakes we made, or the "trials" we went through to grow and heal. Without it would our "hopes of escape" from the hell we made up be dashed into the pit of utter hopelessness.

What Sondra "worked through," and what we all continue to "work through," is the vastness of the subconscious mind that stored up memories of "pain and suffering," which unfortunately replay and take shape again, as most "memories" do. This last account of Sondra's "process" in working through that "insanity" is candid. Perhaps too much so. Maybe it is TMI, "too much information," and even "scary" to some "uninitiated" in the significance of past life regressions and metaphysical "stretches" and restructurings of our soul as we know it.

In this story of her experiences, Sondra was facing her "personal, family, and religious shadows," that the great "hugging saint," Amma, pointed out everyone interested in spiritual awakening has to face in order to evolve and to heal. I reckon they are surmountable, or we would not have written this book. But these "shadows" take guts for us to even admit are there, then take a determination to clear them, amidst uncharted territory that has very few (if any) maps through the pitfalls. This final, unnumbered chapter, "My Most Difficult Initiations as a Healer," describes Sondra Ray's navigation through those shadows. And those pitfalls. All out there in plain view. And her ultimate emergence into the grace of the Divine Mother's healing effulgence.

With utmost purpose, and ultimate "light" dawning, having been willing to face that "dark night of the soul," I believe Sondra's final prayer to the Divine Mother at the end of this account is a masterpiece in spiritual literature. It is as lofty as the poems of St. John of the Cross, or other lesser or greater-known saints who also faced that ultimate Dark Night of divine yearning.

And as the Initiation was meant to usher in the DIVINE MOTHER MOVEMENT in Sondra Ray's Mission and Life, with Whose contact is absolutely essential for *RSH to fully happen*, this account of her trials and ultimate arrival at that place of "surrender to the Divine Mother" stands as the Energy Force from which any meaningful wisdom coming out of Sondra Ray would ensue.

Rather then, not a distraction from the healing approaches laid out in the main body of *RSH*, this "initiation" chapter could be the *point d'appui* from which these insights have sprung forth. The "compost heap of creativity" can have its unpleasant smells, but no one doubts its fertility—rich earth out of which nourishing foods spring forth.

These are my "thoughts" about including this "fantastic" and "vulnerable" story. I feel the Divine Mother is behind it, as She is certainly behind Sondra Ray in all of her Life Actions. And therefore, it would be a *chickening out* to exclude it. "Fear is not justified in any form." (Lesson 240 in ACIM). Therefore, the three of us, Barbara, Sondra and myself, agreed to include this important section of *Revolutionary Spiritual Healing*—in action, as it was and still is in Sondra's life.

It is not a small matter, to leave it in. We pray the Divine Mother will guide you through your own trials to the healing boon of Her Love and Care. We are certain She will give you Her proper and most truthful guidance when you sincerely ask for it. It will be given.

Hugs,
Markus Ray

My Most Difficult Initiations As a Healer

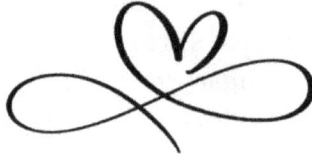

Going Toward the Stargate

Sometimes the challenge of being a committed lightworker is shocking. For example, I never dreamed I would go through a kind of "crucifixion" in France. Actually, it was a spiritual "opening" or initiation, that felt like a crucifixion. I had asked for liberation in this life, and immortality; and I have an assignment to be a pioneer in this life, so I should not have been surprised. But it would be a lie to say I was not shocked at what happened.

I started the journey January 1, 1992. I was aware that the big day, January 11, was coming up, and I should have known I would be profoundly affected. This was networked as a special day, like Harmonic Convergence, for an evolutionary leap. Lightworkers gathered around the globe and linked up to welcome the dove, the symbol of planetary ascension. Under the direction of Archangel Michael, three stargates were to be opened, one at each pole and one symbolizing the Holy Trinity, as formlessness and spirit. This I already knew from the *World*

Ascension Network Newsletters and by word of mouth through colleagues in the consciousness movement. A newsletter stated that "Through the newly opened stargates flows a Christ-like 'super glue' that would serve to hold the etheric perfect to the physical imperfect. It was said that over the course of the decade, and in specific order, all blueprints, grids, and ley lines would be set into place." Fine, I was into it! I agreed to fast on January 9, 10, and 11, and I would meditate at the agreed time, 11:11.

It so happened that around this time I had been instructed by my teacher in Spain to move to France. I was having a hard time with this assignment because I did not speak French and I had a block to learning it. All my guides agreed that I needed to be in Europe during this time to help support these changes. I had always been good about fulfilling every assignment, so I set out for France to tour and see where I should locate. My teacher Shastriji in India had instructed one of my students, Shanti, from Paris, to accompany me. The only direction I received on the phone from a guide was to go to Bordeaux and find a man named Peter. This mystified me. I had no clue where to find him, and everyone said I was nuts for going to Bordeaux. I could not tell one town from another. I knew nothing about France.

Halfway there, Shanti and I stopped to visit some people we knew. I was shocked to see them living with only a fireplace stove. I was *freezing*. This added to my resistance, which then really began building up. I felt helpless as I did not know where I was going. I did get it in my head, though, that I must find the place the Dalai Lama had visited. I had no idea where that was either, but I knew I had to go. The first night we stayed in a delightful town called Salat.

I was so cold that I had to sleep with a fur-lined coat. I could not imagine people living like this in modern times: who needs this? But we found the Buddhist center, and we found a man named Peter there, so I felt I was on the right track. But why did my guides send me on this route? The people I met through Peter started showing us a few castles. They kept wanting me to see these castles from the 1200s. Again, I thought, "who needs this? I am futurist." The more castles I saw, the deeper I went into resistance. I felt forced backward in time and I hated it. At that point, I could not imagine living in France. I was told I needed the astral influences, but what kind of nonsense was that? I felt my guides had not given me enough information. (Later I realized that had they done so, I would not have taken this trip.) Things got harder. The miracle was that Shanti was an amazing Breathworker. She always helped me and translated. Sometimes we would be in a little French town, and we were the only ones in the hotel (always freezing). It seemed that everyone ate goose liver and went to bed very early because there was nothing happening.

Pretty soon, I told her I had had it, and I wanted to go farther south where it was warmer. What *was* my problem with France, anyway? Everything seemed too difficult. I was not used to this at all. I could not understand what was going on. I had lived in Peru in the Peace Corps and had taken Breathwork to Russia and Ghana, Africa. So why on earth was I this resistant to France? Finally, I could stand it no longer. I called my teacher in Spain.

I confessed. I told him that if this was a test, I was flunking it. I told him I could not get my mind together and so on. He informed me that I had a past life in the year 1213 in France and I had failed to complete my mission because a war had broken out. I needed to visit the area of Avignon and St-Remy where I would get a lot of answers.

We had been close to the right places and, as it turned out, we were to return the car to Avignon. I had a very adverse reaction to that town. The popes had gone there once to escape. I guess it was a powerful town, but for me, it was where the hell really began. One afternoon I was walking the streets as my teacher had told me to do. I was looking in a shop window, and I suddenly lost my vision. Everything turned black. I was alone at the time and felt I was fainting. I grabbed a light pole and squeezed my nipples very hard to stay in my body. I was swaying and I could not remember where my hotel room was. Miraculously, it was right in front of me, so I ran to my room and cried. I had enough sense to realize my past life was coming up. I had been through past lives before. Why was this one so much worse? I insisted to Shanti that we get out of Avignon the next day. I could not stand it. I sent a fax to Spain and the fax that came back arrived totally black. So much for that!

We made it to St-Remy. The keys got locked in, so we had to stay. I could not escape this time. But I was quite interested in this town. After all, it was the home of Nostradamus. We headed to the Nostradamus Café to report the key situation, but it was Sunday. This was complicated. No hotels were open for the winter except an old chateau on the outskirts of town. It was very cold. Shanti and I checked in. There we were—the only guests again!

That night I had a very unusual dream. It was the beginning of my opening, but I still did not understand what was going on. I dreamed that I saw a serpent, cut up in pieces. A painter came along, got the pieces, and made them into a breathtaking painting. The painting was so lovely that I could not get over it. It seemed to have been painted by one of the impressionists.

I knew I was going to have to stay in town two days, but I was in bed the whole time. I spent some of the two most difficult days of my life in that chateau, which turned out to be on the property that had belonged to Nostradamus. At that point, it was January 7 and 8. I was doing conscious breathing like mad, alternating dry and wet. Shanti had to take care of me because my cranium began shifting wildly. The pain seemed intolerable. My bones were on fire to the point it was too intense to tolerate. I could not let go of the thought "this is too hard!" and I felt I was going crazy. (Vincent van Gogh cut off his ear in that town!) I cried and cried and cried. I thought death would be easier. I told Shanti that if my mind were to go too far left, I would be insane, and if it went right, I would die. I was searching for a hairline down the middle. The ordeal began to seem like the drama of Faust and the painful struggle to de-throne the ego. I had been through initiations before, I had been through cranial shifts before, I had certainly felt my bones on fire before, but *never* like this.

Then I recalled that Ram Dass said that as you get more spiritually connected, more difficult matters come up. I had not wanted to hear that, but now that sentence was helping me to stay sane enough to begin to recite to Shanti what I could remember from A Course in Miracles, which I had forgotten for the first time to bring with me. I was able to access the lines I needed and that seemed to be the only thing that kept me sane. If I had not been able to recall specific wording from A Course in Miracles and had to rely on religious dogma right then, I would have become insane like van Gogh. (That is what got him—the sacrifice and suffering aspect of religious dogma, it was said.) A Course in Miracles saved me; it and Breathwork. Later I was told that my guides and teachers had all deliberately pushed me to the limits.

I was able to directly experience how my ego could resist a solution—the ego always does. It is like the devil tempting someone to think no solution exists. This part of my mind made me feel utterly helpless. But I kept doing Breathwork. My ego began losing its supremacy, but it forced a huge battle. I finally remembered the part of ACIM that says that the Holy Spirit is the only true therapist, because the Holy Spirit is conflict free. I started shouting, "The Holy Spirit in me knows the solution." And the solution was to keep inviting the Holy Spirit to replace my ego.

I remembered that ACIM said that the ego is insane. I was having an ego attack; but I did not know why until long after the whole experience.

On the third day, I told Shanti we must make it to Provence and get me to an acupuncturist. I could not even sit up in the car. I started sweating and my clothes became soaking wet. I was out of it; but I dragged myself to this wonderful acupuncturist. When I saw him and began striping down, I suddenly took my shirt off and wrung it out in front of him. The sweat in that one shirt made a huge puddle on the floor. I guess I made a big splash in his mind as well, because he took it all very serious after that. I told him I was not sick, but I was having a spiritual opening. He said he could see that. He told me that my fire energy was on total overload. He worked on me a long time and that helped.

After that, I checked into the finest hotel I could find; Cézanne stayed there. At least it was restored and warm, and best of all, I could get CNN! Being able to see news for the first time in months helped me. I realized I was homesick. But that was nothing compared to the rest of the process.

It was January 9. I began sweating heavily again. Shanti changed my sheets every hour all during the night. I stayed in bed for two more days. By now, my teacher Jose, who was monitoring the whole thing from Spain, sent a message that all was well and that I must go through this. He still did not tell me why. He said the energy I was getting would benefit me and everyone in contact with me. But I felt like killing him—literally! He was pushing me too far. It was too much. Did he have *any* idea how much this trip was costing me? That I had nearly gone insane? That I had nearly died and had a horrible time? I felt I would never recover. I was stuck on that thought for an entire day. I felt wounded, permanently injured. Shanti cared for me every second because I could not move.

And then finally it was the 11th, the day they "unlocked the gates of heaven." At least I had done well with fasting; I could not have eaten a thing for days even if I wanted to.

At 11:11, I began meditating. The fire had calmed down. I had stopped sweating; but then I began to cry again. I felt as though I was being ripped open, something like St. Theresa wrote about: "God has ripped me open." Frankly, it felt more like wild lions to me. I failed to see the rapture of it. I could not stop crying. That night I dreamed a man was killed by a wild lion. The father of the man blamed the siblings for the death. I took the siblings into my room and reminded them that they were not to blame. (I was reminding myself that others were not to blame for this battle I had been through.) In the second part of the dream, I was in the Himalayas. White snow was everywhere. Suddenly, off in the high peaks, I saw a huge red circle pulsating. It was fresh red blood. I shouted, "What is *that!*" I was told it was a pack of wild lions during mating. I did not understand that dream.

The day after 11:11, I decided to go to Madrid and face my teacher. I was still angry with him for putting me through this. Shanti had to go back to Paris. In the Marseilles airport, I kept chanting, "I will not faint!" In Madrid, I called Jose immediately. Surely, he knew I was mad at him, because for the first time, he invited me to his home. When I got there, he poured me a brandy to calm me down. He was so loving and humble that I completely forgot I wanted to kill him. He said that I did not have to live in France; just go there and clear my past lives. I could have sworn he had told me to live there. I know he did. But if he had just said, "Go to France to clear," I would have been like a tourist. I would never have gone that deep.

He told me he had to clear me because I had to oversee many healers in the future when great epidemics were expected. Then he told me I was not yet done in France; I had to go to Portiers. I told him there was *no way* I was going back there that year. He would not tell me who I had been in that past life or those lives. Maybe it was better. I felt half dead in his presence. But he kept telling me to connect with the good work I had done back then. I kept dreaming of towns in France burning during war.

The last night in Madrid, my organizer had a dream about the two of us looking at a picture of Babaji. Suddenly, we looked at the sun and that very picture appeared in the sun and became alive. Later we were in the house, and Babaji suddenly came through the window as a huge flame directly from the sun and entered my body. I guess I slept through that; however, my organizer said I was filled with flames from the sun and Babaji was inside me. Then Babaji materialized next to me and began speaking broken Spanish the way my organizer spoke broken English. (Babaji always told us that if we see Him at night in a dream, He was there because we cannot make up dreams about an avatar.)

The next morning Jose called to say good-bye and told me to go where there was sun! He and Babaji were obviously in cahoots over my process! He read a poem he had written for me, something about letting go of the bitter taste of that experience. I did it. But then he said I had to go back to France the next year.

On that trip, I took two female companions with me. Shanti and another gal. When we arrived at the home of Joan of Arc, we all became rather sick and began shaking. During that trip, I was saner and did not have to go to bed so much. However, I needed to see an acupuncturist again. I told him I was in town to clear my past lives. He suddenly ran upstairs and got a thick book on the history of France and started reading to me in French about some king. I thought, "What possessed him to open to that part? Was he channeling? Was I that king?" I cannot remember any of it except that he read to me in French for a half hour while I was under the needles. He was determined that I should know that time in French history. I did not understand what he was saying, but my translator summarized it. At the time, I knew it was perfect. Now, I cannot remember any of it.

After that, I went to India. At the end of my annual trip, I was shocked to have my teacher Shastriji put a tourniquet on my left arm and shout a mantra at my third eye for five straight minutes. He said he was going to unravel my mind completely. Then I went to Madrid to rest, and I was flat out again for five straight days; I could not move. This time I was not going mad, but I could not move. I prayed constantly. Help came at last. A healer from Majorca walked in the door. While she worked on my body for three hours, kneading it like bread dough, she saw many past lives. Then she said I was going to go through the resurrection.

I was scheduled to go to San Sebastian, but I could not get on the plane without help. My assistant that week was a Chinese millionaire. (I remember her wearing Armani clothes in the Madrid airport.) At the presentation, one hundred people were waiting for me. I could hardly stand up, and I was soaking wet again. I decided I was going on stage no matter what. I started sharing in Spanish what was happening to me. Then suddenly I was resurrected, and right in front of them! A frightful loud sound roared through the electrical system as if it had its own kundalini coming toward me. When that blast came out of the microphone, it had such a force that it entered my body, and I jumped. I was healed! I was resurrected right then and there.

I spent the year recovering from that initiation. But that year in India, Shastriji put tourniquets on both my arms and shouted mantras again. I had this treatment three times. I should have known the next year might be even harder. *Harder?* What an understatement!

Initiation into the Void

It was December 1, 1994, eleven days before the important evolutionary leap called 12:12. On this day, vibrations were altered on the earth, new amino acids were triggered in our bodies with new hydrogen matrices, and a spiritual quickening happened, making aging and death optional, so it was said. I should have known something major would happen to me considering what happened on 11:11. But I went ahead with my plans to go to Egypt to join others who were going there for more knowledge on physical immortality. Because I had been there before and had taken a tour, I agreed this time to be a leader on one of the boats. Many other leaders were going, fortunately, because in the end, I did not make it.

On December 1st, I was standing before my colleague's lovely altar in Santa Fe, New Mexico enjoying the essence of Quan Yin. I felt totally innocent. Suddenly, a force from outside my body hit me very hard over the heart area. At the same moment, the woman of the house came down for our meeting, so I did not mention it. I thought it was unusual, but we continued with our meeting, and I thought the effect would go away. After the meeting, I could hardly move, but the next day I was in the car going to the airport anyway. I began shaking violently and Emily's daughter Victoria, who was driving the car, flat out informed me she was not going to take me to the airport in that condition. I said, "Oh, this is just some kundalini moving. I will be all right." But I was not all right. I could not get on the plane. I thought "I will just go tomorrow instead." But the next day was worse. I was in a thoroughly strange state. That night I received a call from a guide in Puerto Rico. She said, "A man wearing white robes has appeared with flowers for you; he is laying them at your feet and saying you are NOT to go to Egypt. You are to stay where you are and have your own private initiation in seclusion." Well, that was really a clear instruction and I had to resign myself to the fact that I was not going to Egypt. But that was not the main problem. The main problem was that I felt like someone had grabbed my heart area and was squeezing it. The pain was almost intolerable.

I called another teacher in Santa Fe for help. She came over and sat with me, and all she told me was that for two years one of my gurus had prepared me for this. It was an "initiation into the void." She said I must go through it alone. She added that I was to open my heart to the level that Gandhi had attained, and THAT was going to be very difficult. She said that I must learn to feel compassion for the whole world.

One thing (besides breathing a lot) that helped me was Rolfing. My Rolfer came and gave me three sessions that week. That made me feel saner. She was extremely supportive. People were very kind to me; but nobody could really explain what was happening. I was able to get help clearing the past lives coming up. But that was only one aspect of the whole process. Again, I cried almost continuously. If I could not have cried, I would have gone crazy. I wrote to my gurus and put the letters on the altar. One wrote me back and told me to *shake out* the fear and that was all. Obviously, I was not to have much information. I had to learn to trust more, and that was not easy when I felt terrible. But at least I was not horribly sick.

During this time, I could not work. I was running out of money. I had to cancel several events, including a conference in Israel. No way could I have handled Israel in that state. Being in such a condition is the worst nightmare for a performer or public figure.

But there were a few things I could not cancel. before Christmas, I had to go to Salt Lake City to conduct an event and then attend an evening event in Portland. In Salt Lake, I had a difficult time on stage, which is unusual for me. It felt as though glass was shattering in my spine, and I felt like I would faint. But nobody knew, and I was able to finish the event. When I got to Portland, I decided to sit down for the whole presentation. Fortunately, the universe agreed and provided a couch for me on stage. I was in a church. I told the people that I must do my devotions in public with them, because I was going through too much. That was the right decision.

During the Divine Mother prayers, I saw a lovely blonde woman in the audience having a "religious experience." She was shaking and crying. I hoped that she would come and tell me about it at the break and she did. She stood in line to speak to me; then she shared that she had seen my guru Babaji on stage with me.

"Thank God," I said, "I need to know if He said anything." She told me He had said that "I had now become the cave and he is taking off the trousers." I understood his message at some level, but I asked her to come and sit with me at the end of the presentation, which she did. I wanted to be in the cave, the womb of the Divine Mother in Herakhan, where my guru had materialized his body. This meant I was becoming what I needed to become! And "taking off the trousers" meant, I assumed, that He was getting me out of the masculine side of my being to the feminine side. Now was the right time, and it was safe enough for me to switch. This switch was one of the most difficult ordeals in my life as a public figure. I had to change at the deepest level. I had to confront every one of my fears of being a female leader. Being a male leader was easier. I had done that in numerous lifetimes before.

At the end, she and her mother came and sat with me. The mother had the same name as me: Sondra. How symbolic! It was amazing. I sat across from Sondra, who just loved me, while the daughter Oshara, a pure clairvoyant, told me the following: "There is a BEING behind you who is like an alien, very tall, and he is holding a long, long scroll of names of women who had made an 'agreement' to allow the patriarchy to take over."

"Obviously to balance the karma of the matriarchy," I thought.

She said that he was telling me I must be the one to break this pact. I must decide if I was willing to take this responsibility. Then he disappeared and she told me I would have to face him later. I took this as another test to see if I was, after all I had endured, still willing to take the responsibility for the Divine Mother movement.

I returned to Los Angeles. In the home of some friends, "the being" confronted me again. He appeared to me one night. He was tall and his ears were different from human ears. I stood up to him and agreed. I woke up in a cold sweat, terrified again. These experiences were over my head. I had to call a friend for help. She kept telling me I was stronger than my fear, which was the right thing to say.

At night, I began to see new blueprints entering my body. It was all code to me, and I did not understand it at all. In one dream, I saw my own kundalini lying on the floor. In the dream, I picked it up and ran through the halls of a university looking for someone to explain to me what was happening. I was told that a professor at the end of the hall knew everything. A very long line was waiting for him. When I reached him, I said, "I only need five minutes of your time." He said, "You can have ten." But then I woke up and did not remember any answer from him.

This was absolutely a process for me to go through alone. I had to get my own answers, and they were not coming fast enough to satisfy me. I had to surrender and trust. It was so humbling, this experience, because I could not figure it out at all. Nor were the answers in any book. I was shocked it went on so long. I grew discouraged and I had to continually choose to live. I remembered thinking that I was having a nervous breakdown, but that was not true at all. It was the death of my ego, and it was a constant battle.

Then I was to go to Japan. I thought I was too fragile so a rebirther went with me, thank God. We were there after an earthquake and one week before the gassings in the underground subways. I went a week early to acclimate. I had tremendous resistance to Japan—probably because of past lives. The little apartments made me feel as though I were in a box. Then there was another major earthquake warning, the very day I was to teach physical immortality to the Japanese! I felt that was my real test. Had I become strong enough to face that without going nuts? I told my colleague that to try to prevent an earthquake, we should move into the heart of Tokyo and start chanting all night. (The earthquake was predicted to occur at 3 AM by a little boy who had superpowers and had accurately predicted a former earthquake.) I called two Japanese devotees of Babaji and invited them to our hotel room to chant with us. I felt the earthquake actually would happen because people had so much fear from the last one that they could have easily created another. At exactly 3 AM, my organizers were in a taxi that was hit from behind and in front at the same time. Their heads were knocked together. They came to the class in shock. The earthquake had happened out in the ocean at that exact moment predicted, but fortunately there were no serious injuries on land. Had our all-night chanting been influential in preventing calamity?

I was going to Maui for the next stop on my tour. On the day I reached Maui, glass shattered around me on three occasions as the tensions of Japan came out of my body. Maui healed me tremendously. The last night after my advanced seminar on physical immortality a minor earthquake occurred there. The couch on which my assistants and I were sitting was undulating. Actually, it was quite sensual. I started feeling I was going to make it.

I now had a long European tour ahead and more terrifying past lives continued to come up. I had hoped I was finished, but no such luck. In Poland, I had slammed the bathroom door in someone's house when a bracket came off and sent me flying across the room into the bathtub. I returned to conduct the training session very shaken and in pain. That was a rough training session because my co-trainer started vomiting after the birth section, and my translator had diarrhea and had to run off the stage. The Polish people, however, were just wonderful. I experienced the power of Poland, and never have I seen so much gratitude at the end of a training.

In Spain, I had the miracle of being able to see my teacher again. He seemed totally aware of what I was going through and could adequately explain things to me. He told me that new channels had opened in me for later work. This was very important, and I had to be willing to "sacrifice for God." He told me that he, too, had ended up on the floor many times unable to work because of the changes he had to go through. He explained that when he was worked on like that, his body would blow up several times in size and then go back to normal. I felt better after that. He helped me integrate the energy. He renewed my confidence that all was in order.

I then took a pilgrimage to the remote site of Our Lady of Garabandal in Spain for Holy Thursday before Easter. I felt I should fast and do penance. It was a long train ride, a long bus ride, and after that, a hike uphill. I had asked several people to go with me, but they could not. Again, I had to do it alone. But after all, I had been to Medjugorje, Yugoslavia alone. I was still fragile but knew this would give me strength. Also, Jose had told me I would receive a "gift."

I was in shock to see what train travel in Spain is like during Easter. The train station was packed body to body as was the train. After eight hours, I changed from train to bus and began the long ride on curvy roads high into the mountains.

When we got to what I thought was a village, I was surprised to learn that there was a mountain we now must climb. I had the wrong shoes and a bag that was far too heavy. I felt critical of myself for this lack of common sense. But I reminded myself that I had been through very stressful times, I was fortunate not to be sick, and I could forgive myself for mistakes like this. Then approaching me was a little man in a pinstriped suit (from the 1930s it seemed) that appeared to have never been dry-cleaned. He was sweet and offered to help carry my bag. We made a funny team, him carrying one handle and me the other, since we were so different in size. I asked him if we had to climb to the top of the mountain, (hoping we didn't) but he answered, "Of course, madam." I found a *tienda* where I could leave my bag, and I bought some tennis shoes in the little village we had passed.

At the top, I stayed for a few hours where the Virgin had materialized. I lay on the grass with everyone else in that precious energy filled with bliss.

When it came time to hike down, I saw crowds of people climbing up and struggling with their breath and fatigue, leaning on their canes or the stronger arm of another person. I saw one woman carrying a huge baby. When she got closer, I realized she was not carrying a baby at all; she was carrying a man with no arms or legs. I wept for his tragic state and her loving compassion.

Later in the chapel during the mass, more new energy entered my body during the traditional washing of the feet of twelve men. I was glad I had come, but disappointed that I had to leave to get back to Madrid in time. A man was flying in to see me, and I wanted to see him. I decided I would hitchhike if necessary.

As it turned out, I saw a man sitting alone in a nice car. I asked him if he was, by chance, going back to Santander. He said, "Yes," as if he were just waiting for me. He drove me to Santander, playing nice music on the stereo all the way. The next day the man I had been seeing for a couple of years came to Madrid. I needed this break. Coincidentally, he had just returned from Fatima in Portugal. We had a great time.

On this trip, I had the great privilege of meeting Mother Meera, the Indian avatar, living in a small village in Germany. I had waited years for the opportunity. We sat for three hours in absolute silence while she worked on us one by one, helping to remove our obstacles. Thousands of people come from all over the world to have her *darshan*. I had been told she was one of my guides for the Divine Mother movement, along with Mother Mary, so I felt it was important to go at this time. The unique gift she brings is to make available the transformative Light of Paramatman, the Supreme Being. She offers a direct transmission of this Light, and she is like a transformer reducing it for us to be able to tolerate it. I recommend her book *Answers.*

Because of this wonderful experience with the Divine Mother, I was able to go on and handle some very tough assignments alone. Previously, I always had co-trainers, assistants, or bodyworkers with me. This time I would do everything alone. In Italy, a blind student had an epileptic seizure. My organizers were out of the room at the time, and I was able to keep everyone calm and centered as the students came forth to help. That occurrence required strength to calm the fear in the room. I had been through so much fear already that I became remarkably calm, although I continued to experience one test after another.

When I got to London, a rebirther did Breathwork on me, off and on for three days. I also needed acupuncture, chiropractic, and Rolfing. I was burned out. But when I got to the evening of my speech, I experienced a power surging through me that I had never felt. There was nothing to compare it to. I was different, so different that I got on a plane and flew to Majorca. In two days, I found a darling chalet near a lovely beach that I decided to rent. I was beginning my new life.

The Last Initiation

I was determined to heal myself completely and permanently and I even wanted transfiguration of my body. After all, Jesus said, "All things are possible," didn't he? A Course in Miracles says the healing of God's Son is all the world is for. I took that to mean, quite literally, that I was here to get healed and totally liberated. It was all going well for me until my mother died. On the first anniversary of her death, I hit a wall. I landed in Germany to work, and suddenly I was unable to digest food. This also had happened to me after my sister's death, but this time it was much worse. I had severe pain if I ate. The situation became grave and then I literally could not get the fork to move into my mouth. This was acute anorexia and it happened exactly one year to the day, after my mother died. I no longer had the sparkling energy with which I helped others to heal themselves. I felt quite literally dead, and I became so thin that my friends checked me into a hospital. My insurance would not cover "anorexia," so I soon lost all my inheritance.

I hit rock bottom and entered the dark night of the soul. Having no siblings or parents took me into a deep depression that was exacerbated by lack of nutrition. I was a basket case, after twenty-seven years of traveling I could not work. I was burned out and I could not go on. A spiritual community started by Jessica Dibb in Baltimore "took me in." I went into seclusion living with a woman named Pat who was like a yogini. I almost never came out of my room. Now I can say I finally understand why yogis go into caves. I call those years my "cave period." Some would call it the dark night of the soul. Caroline Myss, the great medical intuitive, calls it "spiritual madness." She must have personally experienced it because she was able to describe it better than anyone. Fortunately, someone sent me her recordings, so, I finally had some idea what was going on with me.

Carolyn says that after you invoke very direct contact with God, everything gets turned upside down. Your whole life gets reordered, and every false voice is taken away.

She said that you get separated from the world you knew, and you experience a breakdown in the human order. All distractions are taken away and you go into yourself alone and face your shadow side. Thoughts of suicide may come, and you enter the tomb and go through the Lazarus experience. That is exactly what happened to me.

Biblical characters called it the "pit" or the "belly of the whale." Jessica kept telling me one saint was in it for twelve years. I did not want to face *that*. I had no money to rely on my usual healers. I would have to get out of this one myself with her help. I really could not let in much support, but the people in her community protected me.

I had done a lot of work on my personal shadow with Breathwork, but I had not completed the "family shadow" and the "religious shadow". For months I was dealing with the family mind over and over. I even got in touch with the genetics of my ancestors. Then I was dealing with religious guilt day in and day out. I felt so guilty I could not even open the spiritual books that I knew would help me. I felt guilty that I was alive and everyone in my family was dead. So many past lives came up that I could hardly shake them off. Once a week I would drag myself out of bed, force myself to walk to Jessica's, and let her do Breathwork on me. She explained that suicide was NOT an option. (If you commit suicide, you get really stuck on your spiritual path and must come back many, many more times than usual.)

I finally got the nerve to call a medical sensitive on the East Coast. I could not afford many calls to her, but one was enough. She told me flat out that I was going to have to get "off the fence." I knew what she meant. I had very little will to live and had to choose. Only it is hard to choose when you are so depressed. My grandfather had a mental disease (manic depression) and I felt stuck in his mind. I was afraid my brain was taking on his genetics.

It was the night before the turn of the century, midnight 1999 when people thought the great computer glitch YK2 was going to happen. At midnight I finally said out loud to Babaji, "OKAY I CHOOSE TO LIVE." Right then I had an amazing vision. Babaji Himself appeared to me wearing all white. He was standing in a room that was all white. It was a library. The shelves were all white and the books were all white and the pages were all white. He took a book off the shelf and opened it. It was the picture of a brain. Then suddenly that picture became ALIVE, and a real brain appeared. The brain was perfect and totally alive. It was then I knew I could make it!

The next day I began reading A Course in Miracles again, doing prayers, doing mantras, doing processes, and walking Pat's dog, Bodhi. I spent approximately six to eight hours in spiritual practice a day for nine months. In the ninth month, I felt well enough to leave with the support of friends.

Later, after it was all over, I understood what Caroline Myss said: "One has to make a commitment to explore the states on a downward spiral with the intention to experience them fully...like a deliberate descent into an inner hell with the intention to clear one's system. Before the ego can be let go of, it must be known and understood in all its extremes." My Higher Self had chosen this experience and I understood that because, after all, I had told my guru I wanted all that He had to offer.

Carolyn says most people choose *not* to have this experience. It is really for initiated souls who can handle the deepest and the darkest. I was more than lucky that I had chosen to be initiated by Babaji. I knew I had the choice to either check out, die, re-incarnate, and go through another birth trauma, another set of parents, and yet another life of dogma from church and school, OR keep on processing all this out. I decided it was a small price to pay for liberation. That was what I really wanted. If I didn't do it now, I would just have to do it all again in another life.

A friend drove me to see Ammachi who was hugging thousands of people in a hotel. Twenty miles before arriving to the hotel, I felt Her aura. I said to my driver: "Oh, my depression is really lifting now."

When Amma hugged me, it was all over, and I was back to myself!

I did not have much money at all, so I had been kind of hiding out in a cheap neighborhood in Los Angeles. The best thing was that I got over my writer's block. This block had tormented me for three years. It took a miracle to get me over writer's block and it happened this way. One of the neighbors saw me frequently go out and use the pay phone in front of his shop. He apparently kept asking his neighbor who I was. He could not figure me out and it bothered him because he was a clairvoyant. I did not look like I belonged in that neighborhood. Later he told me he thought my mind was like a Rubik's Cube and he could not figure out who on earth I was. One day, he finally came out to meet me. I gave him a picture of my guru Babaji and asked him if he got any messages. He then began helping me a lot! That is how I got over writer's block.

I once again felt the intent of wanting to be the most powerful force of good that I was capable of being. I forgave myself for my former self-aggrandizement of my ego and all my mistakes and I experienced the joy of my own personal transfiguration.

Around this time, I began intense prayers of gratitude, especially to the Divine Mother (the Intelligence behind Matter). After all, I *finally* figured out the secret of all my gurus. They pray night and day to the Divine Mother. Babaji, in fact, had said as His departing words when He took conscious Samadhi: "I leave everything in the hands of the Divine Mother." My guru Shastriji used to pray to the Divine Mother five hours a day!! I saw him do this when I visited him. I had dedicated myself to the mission of the Divine Mother movement and it was phenomenal to be back on purpose after three long years of purification.

I share here a prayer I began reading out loud to the Divine Mother:

> *Praise to You, Divine Mother, You have once again made my life a miracle. I take refuge in Your nurturing arms of compassion. I praise You for once again giving me a spirit of power and love and sound mind. I praise all You have created, and I want Your name to be exalted. You called me out of darkness to your marvelous light. I shout with the voice of triumph. I offer myself willingly to You. Great and marvelous are Your works. May all nations worship You who lives forever and ever. I praise You for Your excellent greatness. With You all things are possible. I am humbled and bowed down as You are revealed to me. You have destroyed the last enemy in me and made me alive once again. You have raised me from the dust and from the ash heap. I sing praises to Your powers because You have revived my heart. You brought me back to life; therefore, I glorify You in my spirit and body. Let me declare Your glory among the nations. I want to always obey Your voice and be Your treasure on this land. You have removed the burden from my shoulders. As Your servant, I will do Your will from my heart. If You will a thing for me to do, I will do it as perfectly as I can and give the glory to You. Let us all praise Your name and greatness.*
>
> *As a newborn baby, I desire the milk of Your word. I have been born again and I love*

You as an heir to Your Kingdom. Thank you for accepting my repentance and giving me victory. You are my salvation. In You, Mother, I have peace. You have delivered me and put a new song in my mouth. I will serve You with gladness. I am lying at Your feet and feeling pleased with the grace of your protection. You are the embodiment of Ultimate Bliss. You are supreme.

You have crowned my life with success and liberation. You are the essence of all that can be known. You are beyond comprehension. You have taken the form of my supreme guru Babaji by whose grace I have been allowed to live again. The love of Your lotus feet gives me lasting happiness. Glory to You, oh Mother of the Universe.

Everything I do is a result of Your Divine Energy moving through me. I wish to express my appreciation to You as the source of all life. You are the breath of life. I am simply your instrument. You are my only goal in life. I desire that all should worship You Day and Night.

I offer up my song to nobody else but You.
I offer up my heart to nobody else
but You.
My heart cries out for more of You.
My soul cries out for more of You.
My life is under your command.

I ask you to guide and assist me in fulfilling the mission I volunteered to do on Earth prior to this embodiment. I open myself completely to You so that I can manifest what I vowed to accomplish during this incarnation. I agree to be part of co-creating the new world with You to the best of my ability. What shall we do and how shall we do it? Show us the way. Ignite us all with illumination.

On finding You everything is found. You are the instrument of the healing of the world.

Oh, that all our actions be that of worship, our words like hymns. May Your knowledge triumph. Teach us all the language of Your heart. I believe You will guide us. Call on me. Show me what to write and speak. Let the words of my mouth be acceptable to You. How can I convince mankind that You are the answer? I will tell the whole world of Your irresistible miracles in my next book, and I pray that everyone will see that nothing is too hard for You. It is you who can destroy the pain of this world. It is due to You that we will be able to release our sorrows. It is due to You that we shall find true happiness.

Show us the way.
To You I give all the Glory.
Love, Sondra Ray!

Then 9/11 happened. I knew, once again, that it was time for me to get back to work. I came out of hiding and started doing free evenings to help people process their shock. I wrote letters to spiritual leaders in different lineages and asked them what we should do as spiritual leaders. The best answer I got was from Tom Kenyon, who wrote that the only hope now was the Divine Mother!

The great saint, Sri Aurobindo, said that the final stage of perfection is surrender to the Divine Mother. In India, they say that there is nothing higher than worship of the Divine Mother. The Divine Mother vibration needs to be emphasized now like never before, since we can see how out of balance we are. The sacred feminine has been suppressed for so long that we have lost touch with our true essence. In each of us there is a masculine side and a feminine side. We are so out of balance that we are addicted to the masculine side and chauvinism runs rampant. Men and women both have been taught to equate masculinity with domination and violence. This problem is accentuated by many religious dogmas. The model of the universe in which a male God rules the cosmos serves to legitimize male control in social institutions. But systems cannot merely be rejected when they aren't working; they must be replaced. Nor would it work to replace the system with the matriarchy.

Historically peace came where the Divine Mother was worshipped by both men and women who ruled together as equals. For example, in Crete, Greece, no one dominated anyone.

When we speak of the Divine Mother, we are referring to the original spark of creation, which is a feminine aspect. The prime creator behind all things is a female vibration. The Divine Mother is the feminine aspect of God, or better said to be the "intelligence behind matter." (Einstein knew this.) All my male gurus in India who I admire so much know this. It is the very secret of their power. We are talking about true power here: love, safety, and certainty, not ego power, which is domination, control, and anger.

When people surrender to the Divine Mother, extraordinary changes take place. When you explore the goddess energy you truly value life. The Divine Mother is the source of all knowledge, beyond everything, and the true release from delusion. This essence of the life force (shakti) cannot be controlled. The Divine Mother as kundalini will clean you out. Your old personality becomes replaced by miracle consciousness. The greater your devotion to Her, the faster your progress. It is due to Her we can achieve true happiness. It is due to Her transcendent nature and personification of intelligence that matter is created. Everything we possess is a gift from the Mother. When we surrender to Her, the intelligence of the whole universe is our teacher. We have the urge to bring forth the inexpressible into manifestation. We remember the ecstasy of being alive! Our bodies can become instruments through which the feminine aspect plays.

Men need to learn to be more sensitive and intuitive and women need to learn to thrive in their own power. Are you, for example, a woman who grew up pleasing rather than being? And do you do almost anything to avoid a man's irritation? Did you immerse yourself in the values of a male-dominated society? Did you re-order your priorities and give your power away just to please a man? Wouldn't you rather be a fully awakened woman with a balanced feminine and masculine side? The more balanced you are, the deeper your relationship can be with all human beings.

Are you a man who is afraid to feel his feelings, afraid to show softness and tenderness? Do you feel pressure to become a money-producing machine? Are you afraid to give up your anger for fear of becoming weak?

Wouldn't you rather become a fully awakened male who is in balance, who could easily channel right solutions and provide the right environment for physical, emotional, mental, and spiritual progress?

What if tapping into the Divine Mother energy in a balanced way can produce regeneration, restoration, and renewal? The Divine Mother has shown me Her renewal abilities in miraculous ways. I had the honor of writing about Her in *Rock Your World with the Divine Mother*. I also have the great honor of spreading the Divine Mother movement in the world to help bring balance to our civilization. It was the Divine Mother who asked me to take rebirthing to the next level which became Liberation Breathing. My prayer is that everyone who needs healing of any kind, can experience the benefits of this Liberation Breathing.

It is no mistake that I wrote this just after seeing my female Divine Mother teachers, Karunamayi and Ammachi. To them, with great devotion, I say, "Oh teach me to surrender to you totally so that we can move forward with this work."

In India it is said that there is nothing higher than the Divine Mother and that only the Divine Mother can give you the blessing of physical immortality.

If you would like a Liberation Breathing session with us here is the link:

bit.ly/LBSession

For more information about the Divine Mother Miracles read my book **Rock Your World with the Divine Mother.**

https://bit.ly/MotherRay

Bibliography

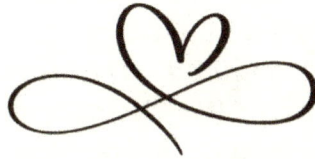

Airola, Paavo. *Are You Confused? The Authoritative Answers to Controversial Questions.* Sherwood, OR: Health Plus Publishing, 1971.

Amritanandamayi, Swami. *Awaken Children.* M.A. Center

Busch, Heather, and Burton Silver. *Who Cats Paint: A Theory of Feline Aesthetics.* Berkley, CA: Ten Speed Press, 1994.

Chopra, Deepak. *Quantum Healing: Exploring the Frontiers of Mind Body Medicine.* New York: Bantam, 1990.

Chopra, Deepak. *Unconditional Life: Discovering the Power to Fulfill Your Dreams.* New York: Bantam, 1992.

Dalai Lama Gyatso Tenzin, His Holiness. *A Human Approach to World Peace.* Somerville, MA: Wisdom Publications, 1984.

Essence, Virginia, ed. *New Cells, New Bodies, New Life! You're Becoming a Fountain of Youth!* Santa Clara, CA: S.E.E. Publishing Co., 1991.

Ferguson, Marylin. "The Paradigm of Proven Potentials," *New Sense Bulletins.*

Ferrini, Paul. *Love Without Conditions: Reflections of the Christ Mind.* Greenfield, MA: Heartways Press, 1994.

Goodman, Linda. *Linda Goodman's Star Signs.* New York: St Martin's Press, 1987.

Hay, Louise L. *Heal Your Body: The Mental Causes for Physical Illness and the Metaphysical Way to Overcome Them.* Carlsbad, CA: Hay House, 1994.

Johnson, Robert A. *Transformation: Understanding the Three Levels of Masculine Consciousness.* New York: HarperCollins, 1991.

Leibman, Joshua. *Peace of Mind.* New York: Citadel Press, 1994.

Meera, Mother. Meeramma Publications, 1991.

Muktananda, Swami. *Play of Consciousness: A Spiritual Autobiography.* New York: Syda Foundation, 1994.

Ponder, Catherine. *The Dynamic Laws of Healing.* Marina del Rey, CA: DeVorss & Company, 1989.

Robbins, John. *Diet for a New America: How Your Food Choices Affect Your Health, Happiness, and the Future of Life on Earth.* Novato, CA: H.J. Kramer, 1998.

Renard, Gary. *Your Immortal Reality: How to Break the Cycle of Birth and Death.* Carlsbad, CA: Hay House, 2006.

Roberts, Jane. *The Nature of the Psyque: Its Human Expression.* A Seth Book. San Rafael, CA: Amber-Allen Publishing, 1996.

Schucman, Helen, scribe. A Course in Miracles. New York: The Foundation for Inner Peace, 1975.

Svoboda, Robert E. *Aghora: At the Left Hand of God and the Kundalini* series. Las Vegas, NV: Brotherhood of Life, 1986.

Tannen, Deborah. *You Just Don't Understand.* New York: Quill, 2001.

Watson, Lyall. *The Romeo Error: A Matter of Life and Death.* New York: Doubleday, 1975.

Williamson, Marianne. *Return to Love: Reflections on the Principles of A Course in Miracles.* New York: HarperCollins, 1996.

Woolger, Roger J. *Other Lives, Other Selves: A Jungian Psychotherapist Discovers Past Lives,* New York: Bantam Books, 1988.

Yogananda, Paramahansa. *Autobiography of a Yogi.* Nevada City, CA: Crystal Clarity Publishing, 1997.

About the Authors

SONDRA RAY, author of 30 books on the subjects of relationships, healing, and spiritual matters, was launched into international acclaim in the 1970s as one of the pioneers, along with Leonard Orr, of the Rebirthing / Breathwork experience. She has trained thousands of people all over the world in this conscious connected breathing process and is considered one of the foremost experts on how birth trauma affects one's body, mind, relationships, career, and life. As she puts it, "This dynamic breathing process produces extraordinary healing results in all your relationships—with your mate, with yourself, and with Life—very fast. By taking in more Life Force through the breath, limiting thoughts and memories, which are the cause of all problems and disease, come to the surface of the mind so they can be 'breathed out', forgiven, and released."

Applying over 45 years of metaphysical study, she has helped thousands of people heal their negative thoughts and beliefs, birth trauma, habitual family patterns, and unconscious death urge which affected their life. She encourages people to make lasting positive changes through Liberation Breathing® to be more free, happy, and productive. No matter what Sondra Ray is doing, she is always trying to bring about a higher consciousness. Recently she has written two new books that are tidbits of wisdom she posted on Facebook for over four years: *Lately I've Been Thinking*© and *Lately I've Been Thinking II*. These give any reader a broad overview of her "comments on the road" and her impressions of timeless wisdom she posts daily to her followers.

MARKUS RAY, artist, poet, and twin flame of Sondra Ray, received his training in the arts, holding degrees from the Cleveland Institute of Art and Tyler School of Art of Temple University in Philadelphia. He is the author of a major work, *Odes to the Divine Mother*, which contains 365 prose poems in praise of the Divine Feminine Energy. Along with the Odes are his paintings and images of the Divine Mother created around the world in his mission with Sondra Ray.

Markus is a presenter of the profound modern psychological/spiritual scripture, **A Course in Miracles**. He studied with his master, Tara Singh, for 17 years, in order to experience its truth directly. His spiritual quest has taken him to India many times with Tara Singh and Sondra Ray, where Muniraj, Babaji's foremost disciple, gave him the name Man Mohan, "The Poet who steals the hearts of the people." In all his paintings, writings, and lectures, Markus creates a quiet atmosphere of peace and clarity that is an invitation to go deeper into the realms of inner stillness, silence, and beauty. He teaches, writes, and paints along-side of Sondra Ray, and many have been touched by their demonstration of a holy relationship in action. His iconic paintings of the masters can be viewed on markusray.com which he often creates while his twin flame, Sondra Ray, is lecturing in seminars.

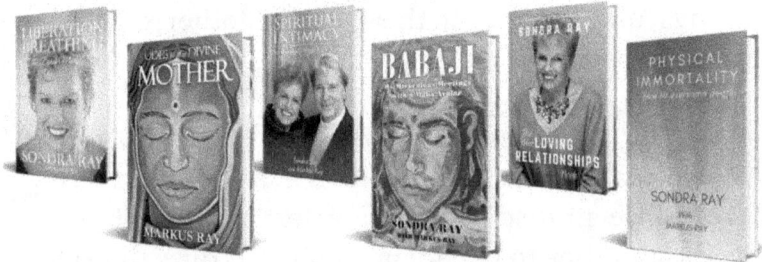

Books by Sondra Ray & Markus Ray

bit.ly/SondraRay & bit.ly/MarkusRay

www.sondraray.com or www.markusray.com

SONDRA RAY'S Author's Portal :

Bit.ly/SondraRay

MARKUS RAY'S Author's Portal :

Bit.ly/MarkusRay

Resources

Sondra Ray /– Author, Teacher, Rebirther, creator of the Loving Relationships Training®, Co-founder of Liberation Breathing®

- ❖ **Facebook:** www.facebook.com/sondra.ray.90

- ❖ **Facebook Fan Page:**
  www.facebook.com/LiberationBreathing
- ❖ **Twitter:** www.twitter.com/SondraRay1008
- ❖ **YouTube:** www.youtube.com/@SondraRay
- ❖ **Instagram:** www.instagram.com/SondraRay
- ❖ **Website:** www.sondraray.com

Markus Ray /– Poet, Author, Artist, Rebirther, presenter of A Course in Miracles, Co-founder of Liberation Breathing®

- ❖ **Facebook:**
  www.facebook.com/markus.ray.169
- ❖ **Facebook Fan Page:**
  www.facebook.com/LiberationBreathing
- ❖ **Twitter:** www.twitter.com/MarkusRay1008
- ❖ **YouTube:**
  www.youtube.com/@MarkusRayChannel
- ❖ **Instagram:**
  www.instagram.com/MarkusRay1008
- ❖ **Website:** www.markusray.com/
- ❖ **"Art Look" – an art lover's companion**:
  www.markusray.com/art-look

301 Tingey Street, SE, #302,
Washington D.C. 20003

E-mail: contact@sondraray.com
E-mail: contact@markusray.com

Babaji and The Divine Mother Resources:

Babaji's Ashram in Haidakhan (India)
E-mail: info@haidakhanbabaji.com

We encourage you, our reader, to attend *The Loving Relationships Training* (LRT) which is produced by Immortal Ray Productions all over the world. You can see Sondra Ray & Markus Ray's worldwide teaching schedule on
www.sondraray.com/programs-seminars/

Also, we encourage you to attend The INDIA QUEST, The BALI QUEST, or other Spiritual Quests that teach and disseminate Liberation Breathing practices, and principles of A Course in Miracles, as well as enhance your Divine Connection to various spiritual masters. These are also available on
www.sondraray.com

Artwork and paintings of the spiritual masters by Markus Ray are available on **www.markusray.com**

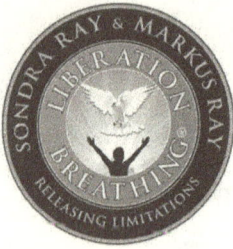

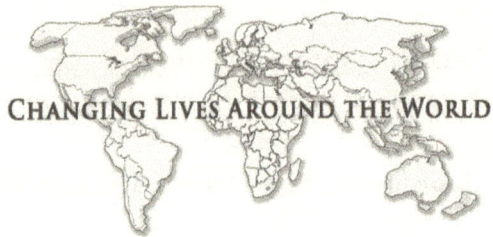

CHANGING LIVES AROUND THE WORLD

Immortal Ray Productions

We at Immortal Ray Productions wish for you to get the most out of your life. Like Henry David Thoreau, we want you to "walk to the tune of a different drummer" and follow your inspirations to the ends of the earth. We help you make this possible. We hope you will join us on one of our Quests—to India, Bali, Glastonbury, Hawaii, Iceland, and new places unexplored—so you will not miss your calling, but rather live your life deliberately and fully, and not wake up one day to discover you had not really lived.

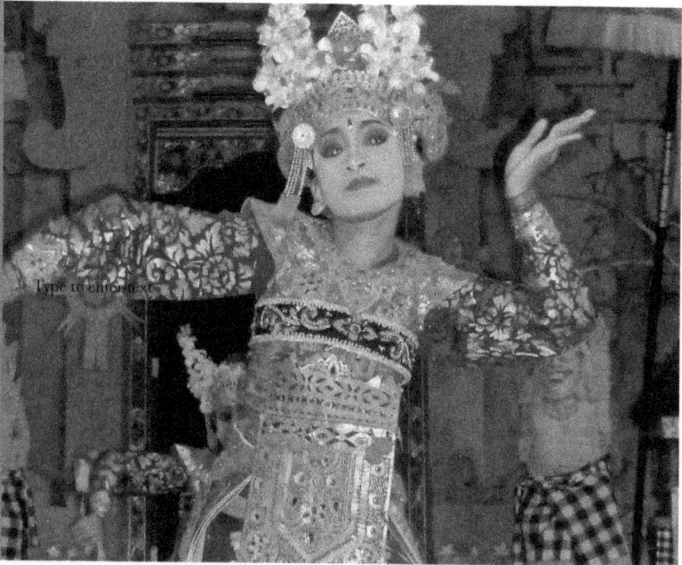
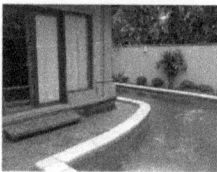

NOTES

NOTES

NOTES

www.ingramcontent.com/pod-product-compliance
Lightning Source LLC
Chambersburg PA
CBHW020524270326
41927CB00006B/438